50 Shortcuts to a Sugar-Free Life

How Pistachios, Olive Oil, and a Good Night's Sleep Can Help You Overcome Sugar Addiction for a Longer, Healthier Life

FREDRIK PAULÚN

TRANSLATED BY GUN PENHOAT

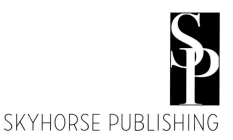

SKYHORSE PUBLISHING

CONTENTS

Introduction

Sugar is the primary enemy for many of us in our quest for good health, weight management, and quality of life. Against our better judgment, we consume far too many sweets, and even more of us ingest excessive amounts of hidden sugars often found in our daily foods. As a result, not only do we suffer impaired absorption of essential nutrients, but thanks to sugar's high GI value rating, we also run the risk of becoming overweight, of suffering from cardiovascular disease, type 2 diabetes, and cancer. For optimum health, it is imperative that each of us be extra vigilant of our consumption of sugar.

This book is written for you, if you feel that either you or someone near and dear to you consumes too much sugar. Its aim is not only to describe the shortcuts that will lead to sugar-free living, but also to explain the reasons why you should strive for this goal.

It is also about my own struggle with sugar dependency, and how I—as a child and then later as an adult—managed to break free from the addiction. I dare say that millions of my fellow Swedes find themselves in a situation similar to mine and that most of them would do well to avoid sugar altogether as well. Today, I'm happy to report that I am nearly sugar-free and am much healthier for it. My weight is now within normal range, and remains stable without any effort on my part.

My hope is that this book will serve as an inspiration to you. Perhaps it will lead you toward eliminating sugar from your diet, or maybe it will point you in the direction of a life free of serious ailments that are routinely caused by excessive sugar intake. You might even enjoy a longer life span after learning how to avoid sugar. I firmly believe that this is my most important book to date, and hope that in reading it you will learn the truth about sugar and the far-reaching consequences of eating too much of it.

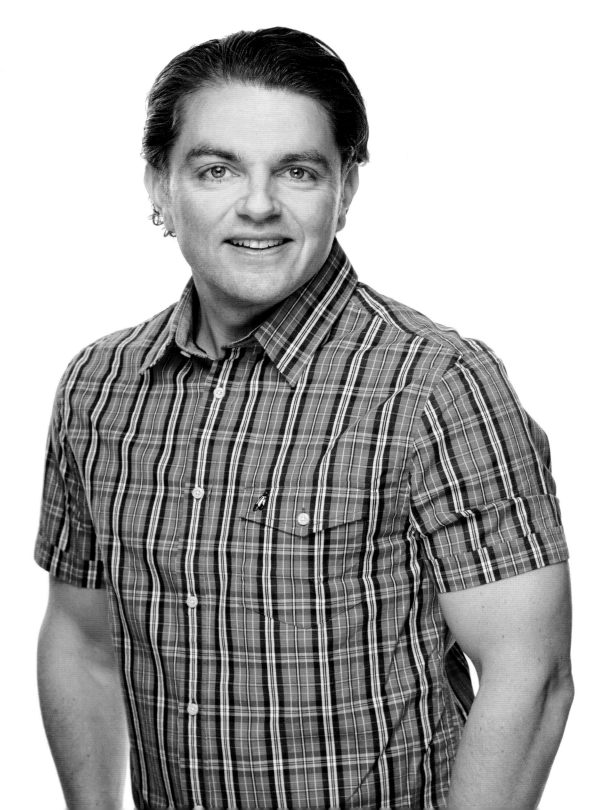

My Relationship with Sugar

Sugar has had me in its thrall for as far back as I can remember. Any time I begin eating sugar with any regularity, I end up wanting it constantly. I quickly become what I call "sugar habituated," and crave eating something sweet every day. In order to avoid being pulled into this downward spiral, I have found it necessary to try to abstain from any added sugar in my daily diet.

Of course, some can easily moderate their sugar intake and seem to be immune from cravings. However, this is not the case for me and many others like myself. Individual disposition plays a big part here. Those who are able to consume small amounts of sugar without experiencing an escalating need for more are to be congratulated. It's possible that consuming sugar carries a psychological benefit for some of them.

HOW SUGAR BECAME MY ADDICTION

Periods of my childhood were very traumatic, no doubt about it. In 1975, when I was five years old, my mother Lena was diagnosed with multiple sclerosis. At the time, interferon betas—modern-day pharmaceuticals that often slow the progress of this particular disease—did not yet exist. In my mother's case, inflammation-inhibiting cortisone was the only treatment available for serious flare-ups. This medication, in turn, precipitated edematous swelling of tissues and caused my mother's appearance to change dramatically; however, the most damage was done by the cortisone's side effects, which included the breakdown of muscle and skeletal tissue. Eventually, when our home renovations to provide a safe environment for my now disabled mother could go no further, she was forced to enter a long-term care facility. By then I was ten years old. Naturally, this was an extremely stressful time for our family, and we all tried to handle the situation as best as we could. I coped by eating sugar.

Sugar provided a soothing balm that lessened my anxiety and made me feel better, albeit momentarily. What I didn't know then—but know now—is the reason why it worked so well: Sugar stimulates various brain chemicals and neurotransmitters in the brain. First, it affects the endorphins, which give rise to a feeling of well-being by suppressing anxiety and providing a sense of calm. Simultaneously, levels of serotonin increase markedly, which lifts feelings of depression. To top this all off, dopamine is released, which makes the act of eating pleasurable, thereby establishing and reinforcing a pattern of comfort eating.

Set in motion this powerful mood-altering process in the mind of an anxiety-riddled ten-year-old, and you can imagine how easily the situation can get out of hand.

THE LESS HARMFUL WAY

Fortunately for me, drugs and alcohol didn't enter my orbit during my teen years, as they would no doubt have inflicted far more damage than licorice and milk chocolate ever did. Hard drugs would have done irreparable harm, had they not killed me outright. Instead, my drug of choice was sugar, and already at seven years of age I understood the impact of quantity on the desired outcome.

Thus, I quickly learned which candy gave me the best bang for my buck; I clearly recall a type of cat-shaped Dutch licorice, because it was fastest acting in its soothing effects. Baking chocolate was another "good value" item; I could scarf down a seven ounce bar in one sitting—the equivalent of approximately 1,000 calories. This amount of energy alone represents half the daily calorie requirement for a ten-year-old child. When my need for sugar was at its most severe, even the Co-op's blue and white melon ice cream would do the trick. It sold for about a dollar for a 17 ounce cup, a sum even I could scrounge up. When I was broke, I would drink syrup straight out of the bottle out of sheer desperation.

On days when there was nothing but granulated sugar in the pantry, I solved the problem by baking cookies. My parents found this occupation creative and admirable; for me this was just another way to feed sugar into my system.

I had no interest whatsoever in exercise of any kind, and was the only student in my class who didn't participate in sports during my junior high school years.

Strangely enough, despite my sugar addiction and my inactivity, I did not suffer a weight problem. Perhaps I didn't eat enough in general, as the sugar dulled my appetite for proper, nutritious food. Furthermore, I grew up in a time before hours spent in front of the TV and playing computer games supplanted everyday active pastimes, and I always walked to school. In retrospect, daily energy expenditure was a lot higher among children during my childhood and adolescence than it is for today's youth.

HITTING ROCK BOTTOM

During my teen years, my family situation deteriorated further and my parents divorced. My new family included a stepmother who, I must admit, became a good substitute for my mother. Meanwhile, my mother, incapacitated and ill, still made her presence keenly felt in my life, which gave me a guilty conscience as I rarely had the courage to visit her. To witness her decline and to feel her empty eyes gaze at me wordlessly was hard to bear. Perhaps she recognized who I was, but I could never be sure. Needless to say, this was a very dark period in my life.

I continued self-medicating with sugar every day, until my father and stepmother found out. In an attempt to stem my excesses, they portioned out—and even hid—the candy. One of my most vivid memories is of a family outing abroad, when during the return journey on the ferry from Germany, my parents bought tax-free candy in quantities to last several months. The confectionary consisted of an assortment of mint toffees, After Eight's, green fruit leather, Geisha chocolate, Mozartkugeln and Bassett licorice. Even today I feel uncomfortable thinking about the sheer amount of candy those shopping bags contained, and the size of the stash my parents hid behind the washing machine.

Unbeknown to them at the time, however, there really wasn't a place where my parents could safely hide the candy from me. Each day I hurried home from school in order to gorge on as many sweets as possible before my parents returned from work, and it took me just under one week to find, and then empty, those shopping bags of forbidden treats.

This did not go down without consequences. My parents, who had looked forward to enjoying some of this candy, were understandably very upset and angry. For my part, I felt so disgusted by my own behavior that it somehow led me to an epiphany. All of a sudden, I understood that what I was doing was untenable and extremely unhealthy. I felt sick to my stomach from eating all the candy and only my fear of vomiting stopped me from regurgitating it all. So while the sweets stayed in my digestive system, I started to clean up mentally.

MY TOOLS

Once a destructive behavior lays you low, there is only one way out, and that way is up. How to head in the right direction is of course up to the individual, but at age fourteen I had no concept of addictive behavior. What I did grasp though, was that I simply had to stop eating candy.

During the first week of abstinence, I discovered that physical exercise calmed my stress and took the edge off of the loss I was experiencing. Equipped with a pair of two pound free weights that were lying around the house, I started doing bicep curls. A set of two hundred repetitions a day was not uncommon. Then I laced up a pair of sneakers and jogged a few times around the block; I soon found that running worked best at distracting me from persistent sugar cravings, and my distances increased until I could run four and a half miles comfortably.

Nowadays we're well aware of the critical role of exercise in treatment plans for various addictions, as it activates dopamine, endorphins, and serotonin levels in the brain in a healthy manner, just as many addictive behaviors do in typically unhealthy ways.

I kept my daily runs up for several years. However, by the time I entered senior year of high school, my body was exhibiting the ill effects of the continuous pounding of running: my feet hurt, my knees complained, and I suffered joint inflammation and shin splints.

By now, I had basically conquered my sugar addiction and the results, both in fitness and aesthetics, were pleasing. As I didn't want to stop exercising it became imperative that I change to a more varied regimen. Instead of running every day, I added weight training, martial arts, and badminton. I still occasionally completed several training sessions in a day; this affected my body but due to the variety in my exercise plan, I experienced an overall feeling of well-being instead of physical pain. I also now felt free to take a hiatus of several weeks to let my body fully recuperate from overuse.

HOW I RELATE TO SUGAR TODAY

My life was often traumatic and stressful during my early childhood and adolescence. Thankfully, this is not the case today and I don't worry about falling back into sugar dependency. These days, the need to calm anxiety and stress isn't as strong, and my awareness of the potential damage from sugar addiction makes me turn my back on the copious amounts I once consumed. Of course, temptation is ever present but I'm well aware that if I give in, it won't take long for the sugar cravings to kick in and become a daily bane once more.

For my body to feel at its best requires a certain amount of dopamine activity, which today I make happen through avenues such as exercise, music, good food and wine, movies, trips, as well as my different business ventures; and last—but not least—through my family and the company of good friends. My life is so satisfying today that I don't feel the strong urge to use sugar as a calming agent any longer.

This doesn't mean that I never eat anything sweet. Sometimes I do, and I enjoy it fully without a guilty conscience. It isn't a problem to abstain the next day, since I know by now how my body reacts. I know that any sugar cravings will be gone in a day or two.

SUGAR IN MY WORKING LIFE

I've been involved in different facets of nutritional education since the late 1980s, and I finished my education in nutritional physiology and as nutritionist in 1995. Early on I discovered sugar's damaging effects and made it my purpose to educate my audience on the importance of minimizing their intake of refined sugars so as to keep blood sugar at healthy levels. I have given hundreds of lectures and interviews about blood sugar, and have written several books on the subject—the one you are holding in your hands being the fourth. My first volume, published in 1999 and called *Allt om glycemiskt index* (all about the glycemic index) was rejected by my publisher who found the subject too narrow. Far from being discouraged, and even though no other publisher showed any interest in it, I decided to self-publish my manuscript. I knew the subject would be of great interest to people and that the book could have a positive impact on the health of millions.

The book was entirely self-edited, as I didn't feel it was economically viable to employ a professional to assist me. (On a side note, I would strongly dissuade anyone from doing their own proofreading, as it is practically impossible to root out one's own grammatical and spelling mistakes. When it was time for a

> EACH DAY I HURRIED HOME FROM SCHOOL IN ORDER TO GORGE ON AS MANY SWEETS AS POSSIBLE BEFORE MY PARENTS RETURNED FROM WORK.

second round of printing of that book, I discovered that it contained more than 200 errors and typos!) Three thousand copies of the book were printed, which I then packed into thick envelopes and dispatched to bookstores, all from my condo's living room in Sundbyberg (outside Stockholm). A few book clubs showed an interest in it, and the first printing quickly sold out. A second printing sold out just as fast, and sales, as well as interest in the topic, have not yet abated. The publication of the book more or less coincided with the stirrings of the sugar debate, and as the current GI and low-carb trends have picked up steam. It was later published in paperback, and a second printing is published under the name *Blodsockerblues* (*Blood Sugar Blues*). To date these books have sold more than 250,000 copies.

I'm also committed to the development of innovative food products without added sugar. The goal is to make it easier for people to improve their health and well-being without having to give up the pleasure of good food. It is a privilege to have been given the opportunity to fight for good health for everybody, and to act against excess consumption of sugar.

What Is Sugar?

Most all of the carbohydrates you eat will break down into glucose in the bloodstream, although the timeframe and pathways will vary. Certain indigestible carbohydrates, such as dietary fiber, pass through the small intestine more or less intact until they reach the large intestine and colon. There are certain fiber particles that are broken down by bacteria into short-chain fatty acids, which are taken up by the blood and used as energy. Indigestible carbohydrates also form gases that you might notice after eating a meal such as yellow pea soup, which is especially rich in fiber. All carbohydrates, apart from fiber, will break down and reach the bloodstream in some form. Below is a list of the most common carbohydrates and what happens to them in the body.

GLUCOSE: Glucose exists in pure form in certain foods, such as fruits, berries, and honey, and also in certain industrially manufactured food products. Sports drinks and energy tablets—grape sugar tablets—are mostly made up of glucose, and therefore provide the quickest way to replenish blood sugar. Glucose needs no processing to become blood sugar and has a very high GI value of 100.

FRUCTOSE: Fructose is also called fruit sugar. In reality, fruit sugar is approximately half fructose and half glucose. Fructose cannot go straight into the bloodstream, and has to first pass through the liver, where it is then processed into glucose. Depending on availability, the liver then decides whether to send the glucose into the bloodstream or store it as glycogen for later use. Fructose's ability to be stored in the liver explains its low GI value of 23.

SACCHAROSE: Saccharose, also called sucrose, is white table sugar, or granular sugar. It is a disaccharide, which means it contains two sugar molecules, in this case glucose and fructose. Saccharose is split in the small intestine into one glucose molecule and one fructose molecule. The two sugars being of equal amount gives them an average GI value of 65.

Invert sugar is sometimes listed on some ingredient lists. This means that saccharose has been processed industrially into glucose and fructose. Invert sugar has the same GI value as table sugar, and has an equally negative effect on health.

LACTOSE: Lactose is a disaccharide identical to saccharose, but made from equal parts glucose and galactose. Galactose is very similar to fructose in both its chemical structure and its function. Glucose enters the bloodstream directly, while galactose is stored in the liver as glucogen, and its GI value is 46.

REFINED SUGAR CONTAINS NO NUTRIENTS EXCEPT CARBOHYDRATES.

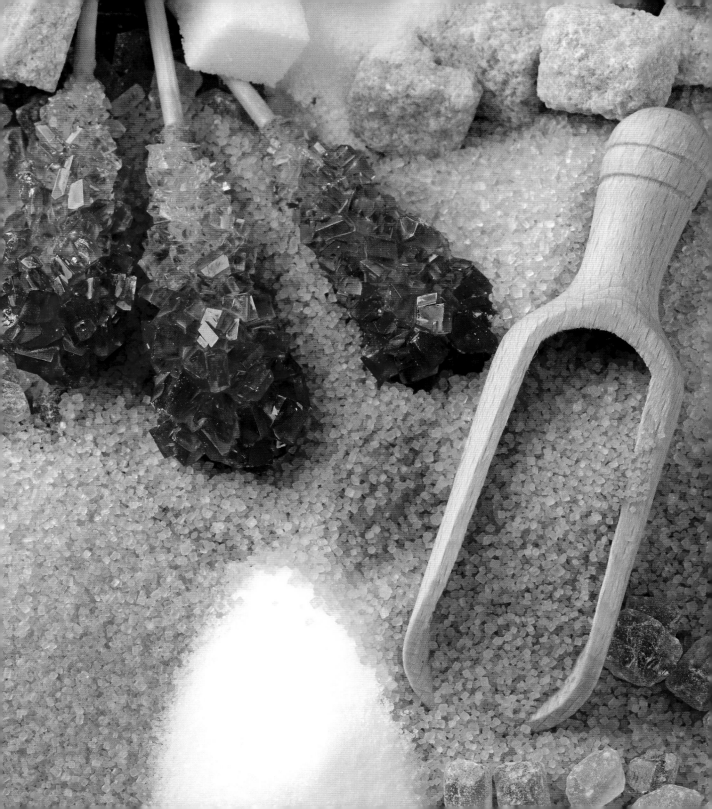

There is no visible difference between low-lactose and conventional milk products as far as GI value is concerned. The true difference between the two products lies in how the lactose in low-lactose products is already split into glucose and galactose. The only benefit of low-lactose products is that they prevent gastrointestinal distress in people with lactose sensitivity—nothing more.

MALTOSE: Maltose is a disaccharide made up of two glucose molecules. Interestingly, maltose shows a higher GI value than glucose. This might be due to certain transition mechanisms for maltose within the small intestine, which makes maltose enter the bloodstream at a faster rate than glucose. Its GI value is as high as 105.

MALTODEXTRIN: Compared to maltose with its two molecules of glucose, maltodextrin is a polysaccharide formed by a longer chain of glucose molecules. Maltodextrin is extremely easy to digest and also has a GI value of 105. It is found in nutritional supplements, it's often an ingredient in weight-gain powders (also called gainers) and is also a part of energy supplements that provide highly concentrated calories.

WHY TOO MUCH SUGAR IS DETRIMENTAL TO YOUR HEALTH

The word "sugar" is sometimes used a bit haphazardly; we talk of carbohydrates, refined sugars and natural sweeteners interchangeably as if they were all one and the same thing. As a result, we lose focus on what's important, and we tend to stare blindly at the word "carbohydrates"—which in and of itself is rather uninteresting—on the ingredient list of a loaf of bread, while forgetting about the sugar contained in the sandwich spread.

There are many reasons why sugar is detrimental to your health and to your quality of life. I'll go more into detail later in the book, but I'll highlight just one reason now: sugar contains nothing but empty calories.

Refined sugar contains nothing but carbohydrates. Fiber, vitamins, minerals, antioxidants, water, fats, and protein are all absent. As the body is dependent on a daily intake of these different nutrients to stay properly nourished and energized, it follows that an overconsumption of sugar will lead to malnutrition.

Even lacking in small quantities of vital nutrients could make you less able to cope with passing colds and viruses, and suffer from decreased energy levels. This is the main reason why the World Health Organization (WHO) previously recommend we only get a maximum of 10 percent of our daily calories from sugar, but has in fact recently been pushing to change it to 5 percent.*

This is in fact a generous allowance, since that translates to 240 calories coming from sugar if the daily calorie budget is 2,400 calories. Sugar is composed of 10 percent carbohydrate, and with its caloric value at 4 calories/gram, the 240 calories equate to 60 grams (2.12 ounces) of sugar. This is a rather large amount, and one that I find difficult to call healthy. According to a report from the Centers for Disease Control, 13 percent of the average American adult's caloric intake comes from added sugars.

Another reason why I personally keep my sugar consumption very low is sugar's dramatic effect on blood sugar and its fat-generating capabilities. I also know that by avoiding sugar I'm better protected against serious illness such as cancer and cardiovascular disease, something I will talk more about later in the book.

---

* Ryan Jaslow, "World Health Organization Lowers Sugar Intake Recommendation," CBSNews, March 5, 2014, http://www.cbsnews.com/news/world-health-organization-lowers-sugar-intake-recommendations/

01

One Week to Diminished Sugar Cravings

GHRELIN—THAT'S WHY YOU CRAVE SOMETHING SWEET

Do you recognize the word "ghrelin"? Ghrelin is a hormone your stomach releases that brings on feelings of hunger, and specifically cravings for sweets (1).

Once it is secreted, it activates the brain's reward center, and sends you the signal that your body wants you to increase its level of dopamine, the neurotransmitter responsible for feelings of vitality, satisfaction, and reward. To up the level of dopamine your body sends you the message to consume what is pleasurable, such as sugar, alcohol, food, or drugs.

Some of us are more sensitive to ghrelin than others. In a study conducted at Sahlgrenska Universitetssjukhuset (Sahlgrenska University Hospital) in Gothenburg, Sweden, researchers compared the genetic make up of 579 subjects. Results indicated that people with certain changes in the gene responsible for producing ghrelin tended to consume larger amounts of sugar than the subjects without those genetic differences. There is also evidence that cravings for alcohol are

CARBOHYDRATE EATERS EXPERIENCE LESS CRAVINGS FOR SWEETS

A weight-loss study compared subjects who ate breakfast containing good quality carbohydrates to subjects who ate a strict LCHF (Low-Carb, High-Fat) breakfast. The carbohydrate eaters showed a ghrelin level drop of 45 percent after eating the meal, whereas the LCHF eaters experienced a dip of only 29.5 percent. This is one of the reasons why a strict LCHF diet often triggers cravings for sweets, and why the diet makes it easier to give in to the temptation of using artificial sweeteners in an attempt to satisfy the cravings. An interesting finding from this study was that the carbohydrate eaters experienced a lower rate of cravings for sweets, as well as higher feelings of satiety than the LCHF eaters (2). In addition, 32 weeks into the study, the carbohydrate eaters had lost more than 20 kilograms (44 pounds) while the "low-carbers" had lost only a little under 4 kilograms (19 pounds).

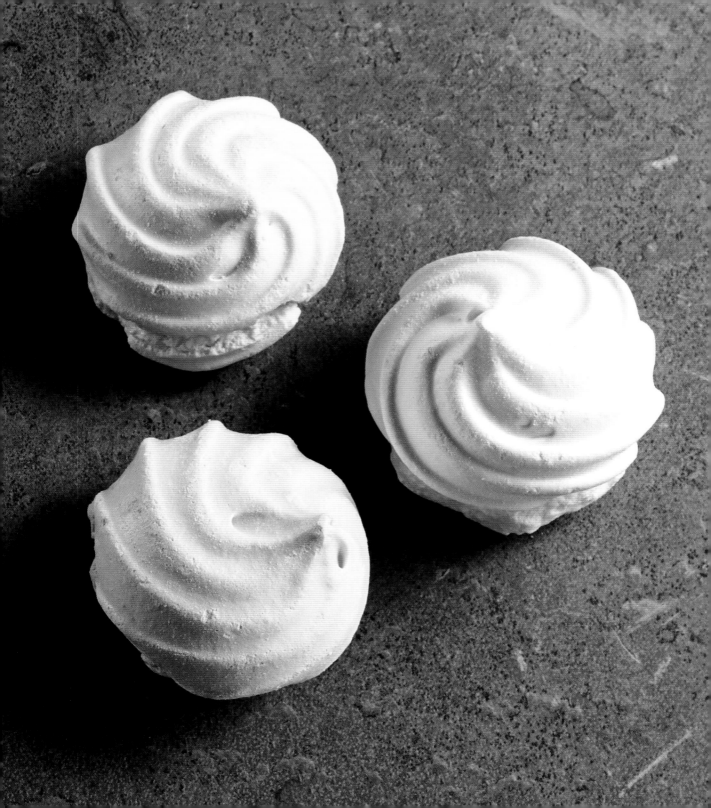

GHRELIN IS A HORMONE THAT IS RELEASED BY THE STOMACH AND IS LINKED TO FEELINGS OF HUNGER AND CRAVINGS FOR SWEETS. SOME OF US ARE MORE GHRELIN-SENSITIVE THAN OTHERS.

influenced by this trait, which may explain why many over-indulgers are drawn to both sugar and alcohol. The vicious circle begins when ghrelin is released and you react by eating something sweet: you establish a reinforcing loop that will lead you to consume sweeter foods to satisfy your cravings, which will make your body release stronger and more insidious levels of ghrelin, which in turn will ramp up the intensity of your cravings, and so on.

RESIST SUGAR FOR A WEEK OR TWO

Some are able to satisfy their cravings for sweets by using artificial sweeteners, and can therefore quite easily avoid sugar. But that doesn't hold true for everybody. As the level of ghrelin increases almost immediately when something sweet touches the tongue, it's common for many of us to feel hungrier afterward. In this case, artificial sweeteners have triggered a craving instead of satisfying it.

Interestingly, after a week spent without eating sugar, the level of ghrelin in the body decreases to levels where it becomes easier for most of us to resist candy, cookies, ice cream, and sodas. I'm sure you have been in a situation where after a few days' sugar consumption—perhaps during the Christmas holidays—you have found it extremely difficult to break free of the sugar habit. However, if you manage to resist those cravings, they will lessen over time until they become negligible. This doesn't mean that you've forgotten the pleasure of the taste of sweets; perhaps the temptation to eat a brownie will overwhelm you at some point. But in the end, it's far easier to resist the call of sweets when your body's ghrelin level is low.

So, resist the cravings! A week or two without sugar or other sweeteners, and the cravings will become far less of a problem.

IF IT'S STILL TOO HARD

Some of us have to struggle even when our ghrelin levels are reasonably low. It might be directly related to naturally low levels of the neurotransmitters dopamine and serotonin.

You can boost your dopamine level by taking part in pleasurable activities such as working out, getting together with friends, listening to music, or travelling. Even little things like drinking a cup of coffee or tea, or enjoying a good meal, will do the trick. A glass of red wine can also dull the edge of cravings for something sweet, but is to be avoided if the cravings include alcohol.

A low intake of carbohydrates or a deficiency in calories will also trigger cravings for sweets. An excellent way to maintain low ghrelin levels is to eat carbohydrates with low GI value, in addition to foods containing a reasonably good amount of protein.

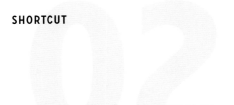

Choose a Natural Sugar

HONEY—A GOOD SOURCE OF SWEETNESS

At the beginning of the 1990s, when I was still studying for my degree in nutritional science, most sugars were seen as being equal, irrespective of their origin. A glucose molecule was always a glucose molecule and fructose was always fructose whether you found it in sodas, candy, honey, fruit, or cookies. Today we realize that this is inaccurate, and that it matters a great deal what else is there besides the sugar. A good example is honey: Honey basically consists of a mixture of fructose, glucose, and combined saccharides, similar to palatinose oligosaccharide. Although the chemical make up of honey is nearly identical to that of sugar, the effect from ingesting the two products are markedly different. Here's what happens when you choose honey over sugar:

● You get a lower blood sugar response from honey compared to that of sugar. This is good news for diabetics and non-diabetics alike.
● Your nutritional profile improves when you consume honey. Your body's vitamin and mineral levels increase when you eat honey, while with sugar they're likely to decrease.
● Unpasteurized honey contains probiotics that support the intestinal flora. Sugar, on the other hand, contributes to the growth of pathogenic bacteria.
● Palatinose has shown itself to increase the metabolic effect of the liver. Because of this, it is easier to keep your weight stable with honey.

The key here is that the honey be in its pure state. Check the ingredients on the label; pure honey should only contain one ingredient—honey. Stores with a large international inventory occasionally sell honey that has been adulterated with both sugar and glucose syrup. This is one more incentive to carefully read both the label and the ingredient list while grocery shopping.

A brand of honey that is either too cheap or too light in color is reason to suspect that the beekeeper fed glucose syrup to his bees (which increases the honey yield and lowers production costs) rather than let them collect the natural nectar.

On the other hand, light-colored hard honey—the most common variety found in northern Europe—is not a by-product of adulteration, but is in its natural form, as there is less colorant in the Nordic nature's nectar.

Liquid honey usually contains more fructose than the hard kind, but the difference is negligible. I suggest that you choose a dark, good-quality honey and avoid heating it too much in order to guard the virtues of the probiotics and keep the active biologic cultures intact.

FRUIT AND SUGAR

Another mistake is failing to differentiate between fruit sugar and everyday table sugar. Of course, it all turns into sugar in the end, but the concentration of natural sugar in fruit is radically different from that of table sugar, and it contains the added bonus of other beneficial nutrients.

This is also the case with dried fruit: The sugars are more concentrated but the nutrients are the same. Dried fruit is excellent for adding a touch of sweetness to breads, muesli, and nut mixtures. There is no need to heed the dire warnings about eating too much fruit because of its sugar content, because it would take huge quantities—the equivalent of many,

many pounds of fruit—to reach harmful levels. Keep in mind also that at that point, it is not the sugar that would be harmful but the fruit acid, which in such amounts could erode the enamel of our teeth.

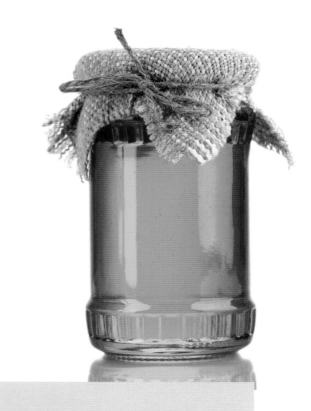

NATURAL SWEETNESS IS GOOD

Certain aboveground vegetables and root vegetables, such as tomatoes and carrots, taste sweet. However, even the sweetest varieties of these foods do not cause any problems, as their carbohydrate content is very low—only between 5 and 8 percent—so it's nearly impossible to eat too much of them. Also, these foods are packed with all the nutrition, including vitamins and minerals, that set fruit and vegetables apart from other sweet foods.

Humans of the Stone Age learned to survive in nature by selecting foods that tasted sweet. Sweetness indicated a non-toxic food that was also calorie-dense. The same rules apply today! Naturally sweet foods add to our quality of life and keep us healthy and slim.

WHY YOU SHOULD EAT FRUIT

As much as I admonish you to avoid sugar, I do recommend that you eat fruit.

Fruit contains 80–85 percent water, which means that it's impossible to consume large quantities of it before the calorie count becomes excessive. Compare this to hard candy, which is made up of almost 100 percent sugar. In chewy gelatinous candy, the gelatin brings the sugar concentration down to 60–70 percent—still an enormous amount of sugar. To illustrate: 100 grams (3.5 ounces) of hard candy is equal to 1 kg. (2.5 pounds) of oranges. The candy contains none of the nourishing vitamins, minerals, and antioxidants found in the oranges, and provides only colorants, artificial flavors, preservatives, and other unwanted additives. While fruit keeps us trim, candy increases our girth if eaten to excess. Furthermore:

● Instances of fatty liver increase with refined fruit sugar consumption, which doesn't happen if fruit sugar is eaten in its natural state (fruit, honey, berries etc.). It's just about impossible to ingest too much fructose through food, as we will have reached satiety long before that happens. Sucrose, on the other hand, produces free radicals that harm the liver, while fruit balances the fructose with antioxidants.

● Fruit does not increase the risk of developing cavities, while sugar does. The risk does not increase with dried fruit, even though their sweetness can seem intense and concentrated.

Dried fruit has proved to be harmless in regard to tooth decay, thanks to their significant antibacterial content.

● Fruit contains important vitamins like folic acid and vitamin C, and is rich in minerals such as potassium. Antioxidant content is high, especially in brightly colored fruits and berries. Blueberries, pomegranates, and the Cape gooseberries are the winners of the antioxidant World Championship.

● Sugar leaves nothing behind in the intestine once it's been absorbed in the bloodstream. This can cause constipation and damaged intestinal flora. Fruit and berries, in contrast, are made up of large amounts of fiber (especially the water-soluble kind), which slows the uptake of blood sugar, lowers blood fats, and promotes a healthy intestinal environment.

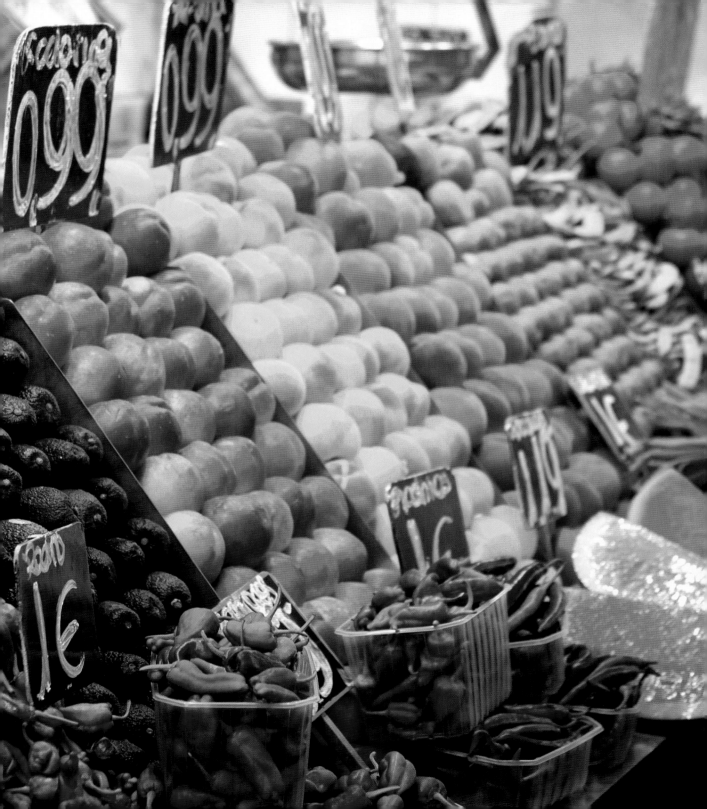

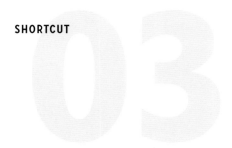

Don't Lose Weight with Candy

WEIGHT LOSS PLANS WITH CANDY

You are far from alone if you have tried to lose weight by using meal replacement powders, beverages, or bars. These ready-made products, with their calorie content already listed on the package, seem like such a convenient solution.

These weight loss aids, for the most part, taste sweet. Why is that? Because they contain sugar, that's why! More often than not, it's not even a sugar-free sweetener (which could, in theory, help in one's effort to lose weight) but everyday sucrose, which promotes energy storage in fat cells. These powders and bars consist mainly of empty calories, which make them useless from a nutritional standpoint. In fact, they might bring on malnutrition if you rely on them over an extended period of time. In Europe, meal replacement products are regulated and by law must provide a specified amount of vitamins and minerals, but due to their sugar content the products remain substandard.

So why do manufacturers use sugar in these dietary aids? In all likelihood the answer is for the huge profit margins, because sugar is a fairly cheap ingredient. Also, by sweetening their products they are tailoring them to their primary target group—the overweight with a sweet tooth—thereby insuring brisk sales. In my opinion, these manufacturers are behaving deeply unethically, and I want to make as many people as possible aware of this cynical practice.

AS IF SUGAR WEREN'T ENOUGH

Another problem with pre-packaged meal replacement powders is aging. Even if consumed before the stated expiration date, the packaged content will have deteriorated compared to its nutritional value on the day of its manufacture. As the powder ages, the protein and carbohydrate content interact with each other and produce chemical by-products called dietary advanced glycation end products—AGEs for short. We have been warned that AGEs are very difficult for the body's white blood cells to break down, and could consequently increase oxidant stress and inflammation.

Inflammation in body tissues, in turn, increases the risk of autoimmune disease, cancer, cardiovascular disease, and diabetes. It is also a powerful factor in premature aging.

Meal replacement bars often contain loads of sugar.

A meal replacement shake or bar now and then probably will not hurt you, but if you make it a part of your daily diet (especially if it is not from a newly manufactured batch), it will most certainly contribute to increased inflammation in your body. Consider pre packaged weight loss food replacements as only slightly better than candy in nutritional value, and far more inferior to real food. The meal replacement products can never provide you with the nutrients that whole food brings to you in the form of vitamins, minerals, co-enzymes, antioxidants, fats, and phytonutrients.

HOW MUCH SUGAR IS THERE IN WEIGHT LOSS MEAL REPLACEMENTS?

Before putting a packet of weight loss meal replacement in your basket, read the ingredient list carefully. If it mentions sucrose, fructose, maltose, maltodextrin, or glucose, put the packet back on the shelf!

Slim-Fast is a brand sold in pharmacies in the United States and the first word in the ingredient list is "sugar." Yes, there are more refined sugars in this product than there is of any other single ingredient. We also find maltodextrin, pure dextrose (glucose), and artificial sweeteners in this product, which will not help any overweight person learn how to ditch the sugar. The ready-to-drink version of the same product also contains sugar, but also pure refined fructose and high fructose corn syrup (HFCS), an unhealthy ingredient known for its fattening and pro-diabetic properties. Kellogg's Special K Protein bar is not much better. It contains refined sugar, barley malt syrup, fructose, and dextrose, which will not persuade me to eat it if I wanted a protein boost instead of a sugar rush. Even products from the product line South Beach Diet are made with refined sugars. Their meal bars have sugar, dextrose, and lactose on their ingredient list. If you want to lose weight in a healthy way and fight your sugar addiction, I strongly suggest that you read the ingredient list and never buy a weight loss product containing refined sugars. Buy better products or just eat whole food. Sugar-free food made from real unrefined ingredients are safe, healthy, and satisfying.

Stay away from meal replacement products crammed with sugars. They have little nutritional value and will negatively impact your health.

These products are counterproductive in the long run, as they keep cravings for sweets alive—those same cravings that might have been the root cause of you being overweight to begin with. No, the only way to lose the surplus weight for good is to eat real food made from real ingredients, and to eat your fill of them to keep cravings for sweets at bay. Combine this with a reasonable amount of exercise, and you will lose weight and keep it off.

THE DRAWBACKS OF ADDED SUGAR IN WEIGHT LOSS PRODUCTS

- Inferior nutritional value
- Keeps cravings for sweets alive by promoting high levels of ghrelin
- Increases insulin response, which promotes lipogenesis
- Supplies a large amount of refined fructose, a sugar that has proven to be even more fat promoting than comparable amounts of glucose
- Likely to sabotage the weight loss efforts of someone fighting a sugar dependency.
- The products taste like candy, which might make the consumer eat more than the recommended quantity.

04

Sweetened Bread or GI Bread?

WHY IS THERE SUGAR IN THE BREAD?

Why we add sugar to bread is a riddle to me. If you want to indulge in something sweet it makes more sense to grab a piece of cake or a sweet roll. Bread is something filling, nourishing, and wholesome. Sugar, with its empty calories, is the exact opposite.

There is only one logical reason to add sugar to bread, and that is as a catalyst for the yeast during baking. Sugar feeds the yeast and helps to proof the dough. Sometimes the yeast is fully consumed by the baking process, and when that's the case the manufacturer isn't required to list sugar among its ingredients. However, far too much bread has remnants of sugar that has not been baked out of it during manufacturing. Sugar can be found in all breads, from buns to syrupy ethnic loaves, rye breads to health food loaves.

Since sugar is a totally unnecessary ingredient in bread, I suggest we show no tolerance when we find it among the ingredients. If the label lists sugar—inverted sugar, glucose syrup, syrup, or fructose syrup—simply choose another kind of bread. Bread made with sugar has a higher GI value and has a less nutritious profile than bread baked with only flour, salt, and water.

"OF WHICH SUGARS"

"Sugar" is a common term found under "carbohydrate" on the bread wrapper's nutrition label. This is meant to show how much sugar is in the bread, but the problem is that it gives us no idea whether the sugar is refined or if it is in its natural form as part of the fruit, berry, or grain used to make the bread. If the sugars are in their natural form, then they are in no way a health risk, as they are accompanied by fibers and other vital nutrients that make whole grain products and fruit healthy and wholesome.

When the label says "sugar" it only tells us how much sugar was added to the product! There is no surefire way of finding out just how much of the bread is refined sugar, and if this is something we need to worry

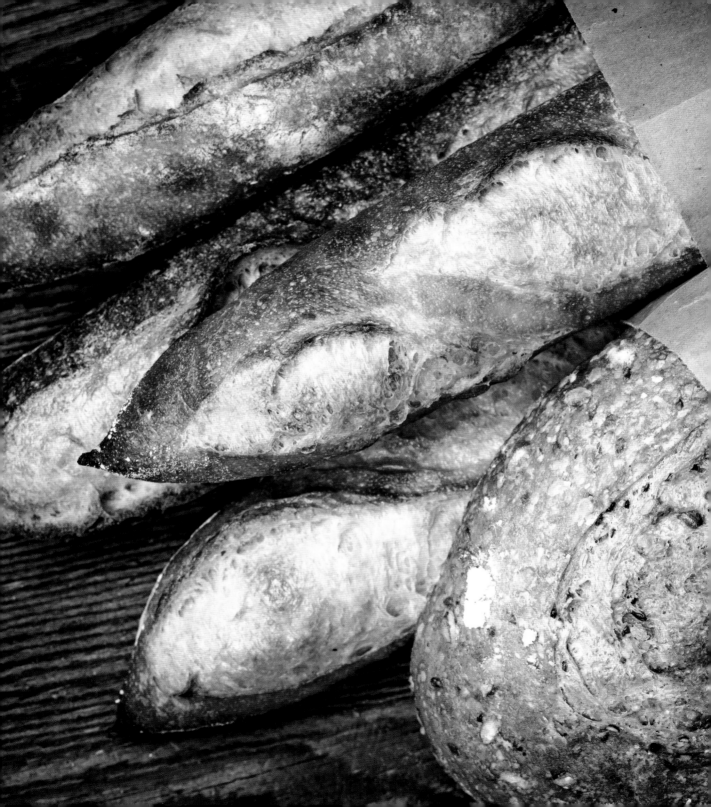

about. I believe we ought to have a new way of labeling food, where the nutrition breakdown must state: "added sugars."

THE PERFECT LOAF OF BREAD

The perfect loaf would be bread free of added sugars, baked using a high percentage of whole meal flour and with added grains, seeds, and nuts. My favorite loaves often have a crust covered with different types of seeds, sunflower for example. It makes them pleasing to look at as well as delicious to eat, and they boast both a low GI value and a high nutritional profile. Compared to refined flour, whole meal flour often contains between 50 to 100 percent more of many vitamins and minerals, and its level of antioxidants is substantially higher.

Sourdough is another great type of bread. It slows down digestion and the rate at which sugar enters the bloodstream, so has a lower GI value. As a result, you feel full longer and get a balanced blood sugar level. Adding fat to the bread will produce the same effect, but

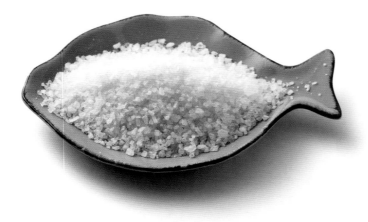

it must to be a good quality polyunsaturated fat such as that found in colza (canola oil).

BAKE YOUR OWN BREAD

It's a smart move to bake your own bread if you have trouble finding good products at your local bakery or grocery store. You have complete control over the ingredients, and you can shape the bread any way that suits your fancy—bake it in tins, or in the shape of baguettes, rolls, or loaves. To be sure, baking requires a bit of time and practice, but you'll save a lot of money, and it brings so much pleasure and satisfaction when the end result is perfect. If you choose to make sourdough, the bread will stay fresher longer, and what you don't eat freshly baked can always be tightly wrapped and stored in the freezer.

For variety, try adding legumes or root vegetables (a good example is grated carrots) to your loaves, which helps lower the calorie content and increase the antioxidant profile.

Chopped nuts are another nice addition ; they change the composition of the bread by lessening the amount of carbohydrates, and raising fat and protein levels.

It's worth trying out the increasingly popular coconut and almond flours if you want to avoid traditional grains. Baking methods will change slightly if using other flours than wheat based, but it is still possible to bake not only delicious breads, but to make those breads healthier by lowering their carbohydrate content.

As a salt source, mineral salt is preferable because it contains less sodium and more potassium than refined table salt. Sea salt is also a good choice, as it provides trace elements like iodine and selenium.

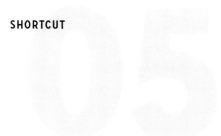

How Sugar Acts on the Body

GLYCATION

As I mentioned in the introduction of this book, a regularly elevated consumption of sugar will lower one's overall nutritional profile, since sugar is made up of empty calories lacking all nutrients except for simple carbohydrates. There are, however, several other issues that can arise when we choose to eat too many sweet things. One of the lesser known yet more serious problems is glycation.

Glycation occurs when glucose molecules in the blood attach themselves to protein molecules and form bonds that are difficult to break down. These bonds carry different names—one is advanced glycated end products (abbreviated as AGE), another is Maillard products—but the negative health effects caused by the damaged proteins are the same in both cases.

AGE is the browned surface that forms on a fried pancake or the crust on a freshly baked loaf of bread. AGEs provoke inflammation, and are therefore directly linked to adverse health conditions like pain and allergies. A high level of inflammation in the body also increases the risk factor for serious illnesses like cancer, cardiovascular disease, and a number of autoimmune disease such as ulcerous colitis, Crohn's disease, type 1 diabetes (DT1), and rheumatic diseases.

Even the process itself of protein glycation leads to many of the problems we associate with aging: stiffness, decreased vision, high blood pressure, type 2 diabetes, and cardiovascular disease (see page 34).

DENTAL CAVITIES

During my childhood in Sweden in the 1970s, we were taught that two small tooth goblins lived in the mouth. They were called Karius and Baktus, and were responsible for our dental cavities. These imaginary fellows—aptly named after the bacteria that exist in the oral cavity—and their fable served to illustrate to us kids that bacteria are in fact real and responsible for tooth decay. Indeed, while a tooth troll is pure fiction, bacteria are anything but.

The wrong oral bacterial flora will often lower the mouth's pH, which can cause a type of damage

RAISINS DO NOT CAUSE CAVITIES, EVEN THOUGH WE ARE OFTEN TOLD OTHERWISE.

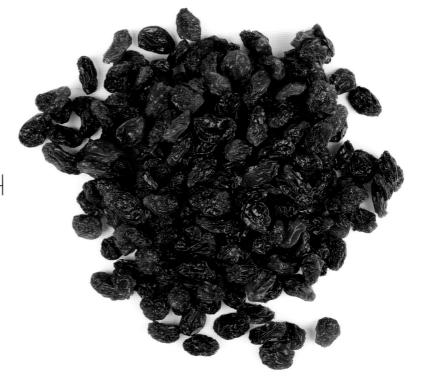

to the teeth known as cavities. A cavity starts out as a small indentation in the tooth enamel; then, as bacterial acids go to work, it can grow into a deeper and often painful hole.

There are several ways to prevent cavities. The most common method is, of course, to remove the bad bacteria and all the food remnants they feed on, by brushing the teeth. Another way is to consume probiotics.

Probiotics are beneficial bacteria that can keep the cariogenic (and cavity forming) bacteria at bay. Probiotics exist in tablet form, but to get full benefit it is advisable to use the powdered form or to take them as liquid drops orally. Some brands of chewing gum also contain probiotics.

If using capsules as a preventative measure, open them and let the liquid touch the surface of the mouth to establish the beneficial bacterial flora directly on the site.

Swallowing the capsules whole is beneficial for the stomach's bacterial flora, and this is probably the most common reason for taking probiotics. The beneficial bacteria improve digestion and strengthen the immune system.

One last, but also effective, method to prevent cavities is to avoid sugar altogether. It is a known fact that refined wheat bread, instant mashed potatoes, cookies, and other easily digested starch-rich foods can cause cavities, but even here sugar stands out as a major culprit.

Remember that dried fruit—raisins, per say—do not produce cavities, even though we have been told otherwise. Raisins are both sweet and tend to stick to the teeth's surface, but they do not increase the cariogenic bacterial flora due to their high levels of antibacterial compounds that work against cavity formation.

OXIDATION—BAD FOR YOUR CAR AND BAD FOR YOU

Oxidation—taste that word. It means something that is affected by oxygen is breaking down.

Rust on a car is a very common example of oxidation. But oxidation is also visible on top of a cozy Friday night's bowl of guacamole, as its surface turns brown and unappetizing because you forgot to add lemon juice to the dip. Lemon's high concentration of vitamin C works as an antioxidant, which preserves the avocado's fresh green color.

Oxidation in the body means, chemically speaking, that free radicals that form naturally in the air around us and enter our bodies via breathing, steal electrons from lipids or from our DNA. The damage done to the lipids prevents them from being fully functional. If the lipids are part of a cell membrane, the damage is inflicted on the membrane and consequently, the cell's function is impaired. In a worst-case scenario, several lipids are involved and the damage is ongoing over a prolonged period of time, whereby the affected cell dies or turns cancerous.

Antioxidants are compounds that scavenge and neutralize free radicals, rendering them harmless. As much as we'd like to, it's impossible to completely avoid free radicals, since after all, we need to breathe in order to survive. As antioxidants are our allies in the fight against the free radicals, problems tend to surface when we don't have enough antioxidants in our bodies. One reason for this deficiency might be the body's inability to produce enough of them. The body produces antioxidants, but in order to do so optimally it needs the right raw material to work with—in this case proteins and minerals. If these vital nutrients are missing, the production of antioxidants suffers and the body will be more at risk of being damaged by free radicals. Someone who consumes a diet full of refined foods and large amounts of empty calories in the form of sugar will be lacking in antioxidants.

Antioxidants are abundant in foods such as fruit (even fruit juices), berries, vegetables, spices, herbs, eggs, salmon, whole grains, and cereals (porridge oats and muesli).

If your diet doesn't include these foods, you will be missing a serious amount of antioxidants, and you will have too many free radicals. Sugar is one of the worst dietary substances there is, because it produces excess free radicals at an alarming rate through its large calorie content. Through digestion alone, sugar causes the proliferation of free radicals, and ingesting more calories means a larger production and more sustained exposure to free radicals. In a nutshell, sugar overpowers and consumes the antioxidants needed to neutralize the free radicals.

Bread baked from refined flours, and other easily digestible foods, can cause cavities.

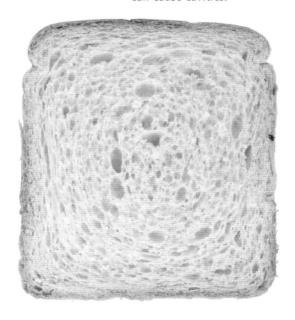

ANTIOXIDANTS ARE PRESENT IN FOODS WE THINK OF AS **WHOLESOME**, EXAMPLES OF WHICH ARE FRUITS, BERRIES, VEGETABLES, LEGUMES, NUTS, SEEDS, ROOT VEGETABLES, **SPICES**, HERBS, EGGS, SALMON, WHOLE GRAINS, AND CEREALS (PORRIDGE OATS AND MUESLI).

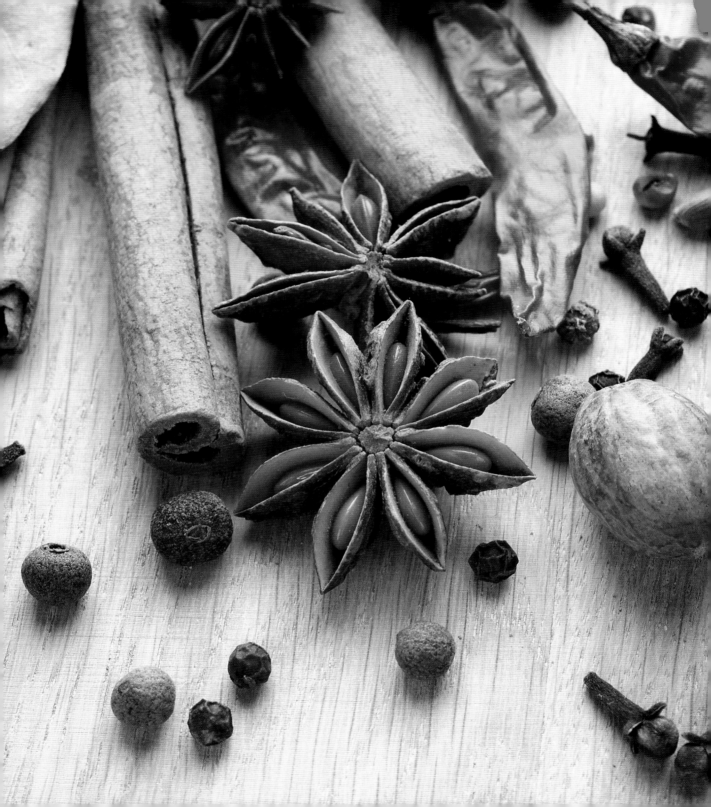

06

How to Find the Right Breakfast Cereals

A CEREAL PRIMER

Many people eat some form of cereal at breakfast or as a snack, even occasionally for a quick lunch or dinner. This is not in itself a bad habit, as long as we choose a wholesome cereal. The problem lies in the proliferation of sugar-laden products. And while it's easy to avoid the many types of glazed and sugar-frosted flakes, it can be challenging to root out the brands that bake sugar right into the cereal grains.

Did you know that Kellogg's Corn Flakes contains 8 percent added sugar, Kellogg's Special K Multigrain 15 percent, and Kellogg's All-Bran Regular 16 percent? Malt is a common ingredient here and we absolutely need to avoid it, because in these cereals it takes the form of maltose, one of the most rapidly absorbed sugars we know of.

So if you want to eat breakfast cereal, go ahead—but you'll need to read the ingredient list carefully and be picky. The following is a short cereal primer covering some of the most common cereal brands on the market:

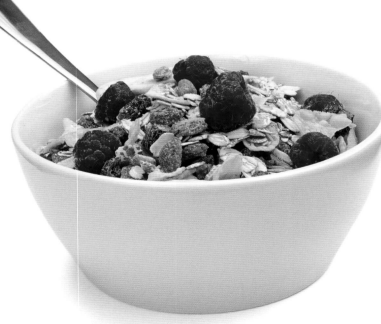

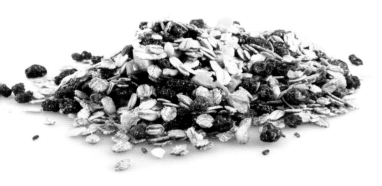

Muesli

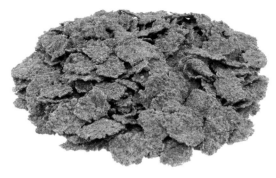

Bran Flakes

THE MOST COMMON BREAKFAST CEREALS

MUESLI: A common name for cereals most often associated with wholesomeness.

If you choose to make your own muesli at home, you can select a myriad of wholesome ingredients such as oat flakes, rye flakes, buckwheat flakes, nuts, seeds, dried fruit, and spices. A nice touch is to roast the flakes before adding the dried fruit. This makes the muesli both tastier and more digestible. Store-bought muesli often contains far too much sugar, something I find rather peculiar. Imagine you have prepared a nice big bowl of tasty and wholesome muesli from scratch and then, as a last touch, you mix in almost 200 ml. (13.5 tablespoons) of sugar! Stay away from the sugary muesli, and opt instead for a small cookie on your coffee break, if you still feel like eating something sweet.

PUFFED CEREAL: There are different types of puffed cereal; some are made from rice, some from wheat, and others are based on a variety of other ingredients. On a molecular level, however, they're all mostly comprised of fast-acting simple carbohydrates, as they are seldom made from whole grains. This means that they are nutritionally comparable to pure sugar.

Instead, seek out puffed cereal made from whole grains such as quinoa or amaranth. Their GI values are lower and their nutritional profiles make them healthier.

Avoid at all cost the sugar-laden and frosted puffed cereal called Sugar Puffs, which is made from refined wheat. Nutritionally this cereal ranks close to candy, and should only be treated as such.

BRAN FLAKES: Similar to corn flakes but made from whole grains, hence nutritionally superior.

31

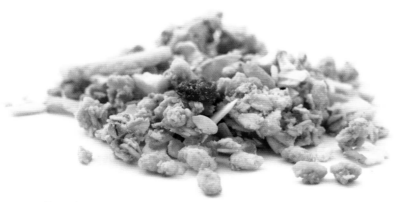

Granola

Bran flakes are usually manufactured from whole grain flour, but watch out: some manufacturers do add sugar to their products.

Unsweetened bran flakes are a better option, and constitute a wholesome breakfast cereal. You can improve it further by adding fruit, berries, and spices like cinnamon or cardamom.

GRANOLA: In Sweden, where this cereal has become very popular, it goes by the name Start! Known internationally under its trade name, Granola, it has become the poster child for unhealthy cereal. Nutritionally, we can liken Start! to cookie crumbs due to its high sugar content and inferior quality fats. Not long ago this cereal contained trans fats, but fortunately we have since passed legislation that prohibits the use of these unhealthy fats in processed foods. Although there are several other inferior granola products on the market—names like Crunch come to mind—there has been an improvement among most brands toward more wholesome granolas.

A nutritious granola should be based on whole grains that are oven roasted at low temperature, and mixed together with some form of soluble carbohydrate to produce a crunchy consistency. In certain granolas this means use of apple juice or oligo-fructose (also know by the name inulin—not insulin). Inulin consists of a chain of fructose molecules that cannot be broken down in the small intestine. Due to its natural properties, oligo-fructose acts as a source of fiber, and thereby lowers the GI value. If granola is made this way and complemented with dried fruit, it becomes a nutritious alternative to, say, bran flakes.

WHAT TO EAT WITH BREAKFAST CEREALS

Consumers of cereal typically prefer—and stick to—three common preferences: milk; Swedes enjoy *filmjölk*, which is a type of fermented milk similar in taste to buttermilk; and yogurt.

As in everything, there are good and bad choices in the dairy aisle; perhaps the most important option is the one that is most ecologically sound. Organic dairy products tend to be more nourishing than their conventional counterparts, as they contain superior quality fats. Also, plain dairy foods should prevail over flavored varieties, as the latter products almost always have sugar added to them.

I choose mild, plain yogurts with 3 to 4 percent fat. It's delicious and the uptake is slow, so satiety, alertness, and blood glucose levels are optimized. My workday typically begins at 8 a.m., so I can easily ward off hunger pangs until lunchtime, if I start off with a breakfast of yogurt and unsweetened muesli.

The same applies for buttermilk: plain, organic, and low in fat is optimal. Oat milk, soy milk, rice milk, and almond milk are all suitable alternatives to dairy for those who are lactose intolerant, or for those who wish to forgo dairy products entirely. Again, read the ingredient labels carefully: even here you will find that many non dairy milks contain sugar and/or maltodextrin.

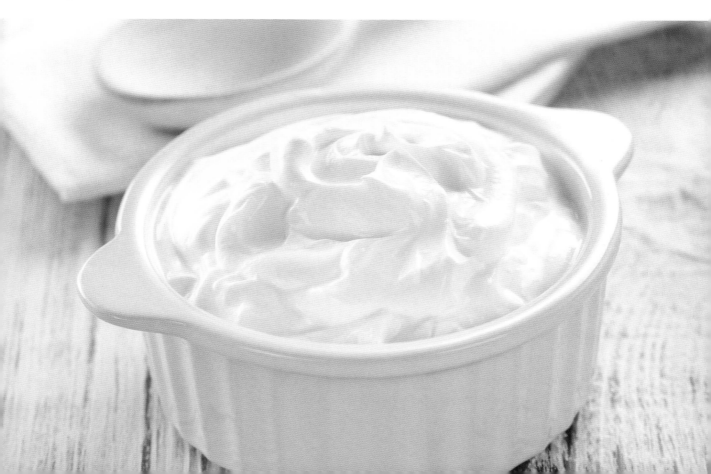

07

Sugar and the Heart

HIGHLY ELEVATED BLOOD GLUCOSE CAN LEAD TO A HEART ATTACK

There are several risk factors for cardiovascular disease. High blood pressure, elevated LDL (low-density lipoprotein—commonly referred to as the "bad cholesterol"), and elevated lipid levels are the most widely known. Often one or two of these characteristics are found in someone who has experienced a heart attack, but there is only one that is present in nearly all cases, and that is elevated blood sugar. Consequently, we stand to benefit from checking for refined sugar in our food to avoid raising our blood sugar unnecessarily and jeopardizing our heart health.

A high level of blood sugar leads to elevated blood pressure, but it wreaks havoc first by damaging the LDL. High blood sugar can damage even normal levels of LDL by causing glycation.

As we saw earlier, glycation is a process whereby a sugar molecule binds to LDL cholesterol and makes it sticky. The LDL attaches itself to the walls of blood vessels, which then become narrower and narrower. This constriction of the vessels causes vascular cramp, and in a worst-case scenario can lead to a clot that brings about a heart attack. If the clot is situated in a vessel that supplies the heart with blood, there will be a lack of oxygen that kills off part of the heart

GLYCATION IS THE PROCESS WHEREBY SUGAR MOLECULES STICK TO THE INSIDE OF BLOOD VESSELS, MAKING THEM NARROWER AND NARROWER. THIS CAN LEAD TO VASCULAR SPASM, BLOOD CLOT, AND HEART ATTACK.

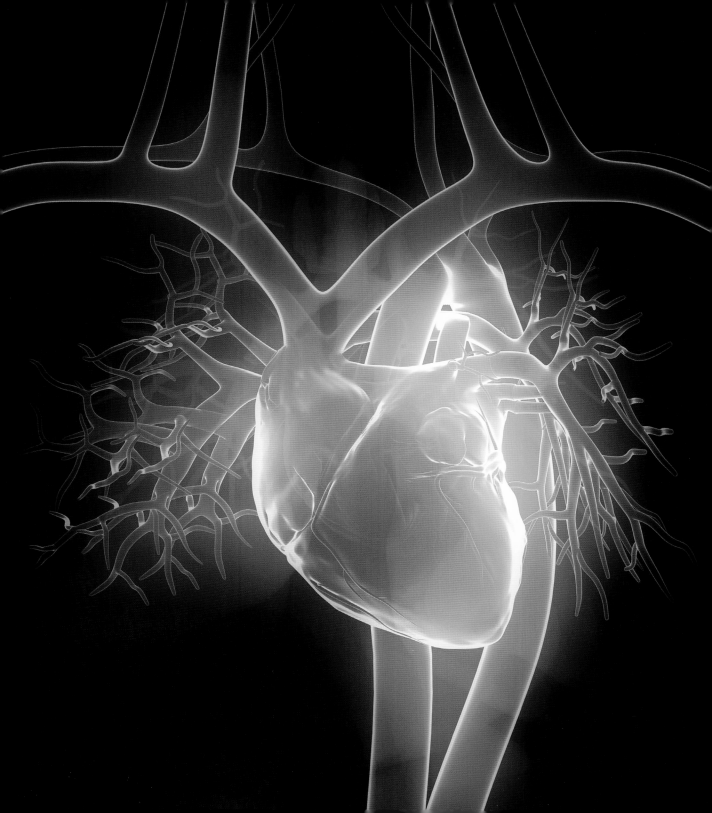

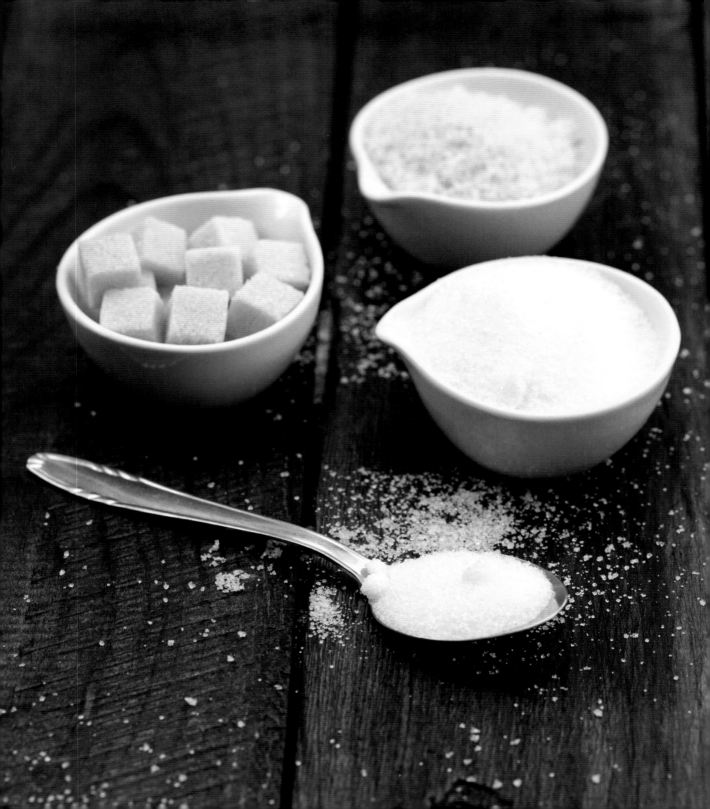

muscle. This can lead to painful and protracted illness, or can be fatal.

Living a sugar-free life is simple; a greatly reduced risk of heart disease illustrates that it is also incredibly powerful.

SUGAR AND FREE RADICALS

Research shows that excessive consumption of sugar immediately increases the body's level of free radicals. There is no way we can avoid free radicals altogether, as they form when we process the oxygen we breathe; also, the more calories we eat, the more oxygen we need to process and digest the food. Free radicals attack lipids, protein, and DNA, and cause damage even to the LDL. Here we see another correlation between cardiovascular disease and sugar consumption.

A big bag of candy will inevitably increase the level of oxidized LDL. If that bag of candy is an occasional treat it might not matter very much in the long run, but if you repeatedly indulge your sweet tooth the outcome will be an increased risk factor for cardiovascular disease.

SUGAR AND BLOOD LIPIDS

Sugary foods have also shown to increase blood lipids known as triglycerides, which are produced by the liver when it takes a hit of sugar in the form of fructose. If the body can't use up all the fructose, the excess is converted to fat, which in turn causes the level of blood lipids to rise. Research shows that it's only triglycerides that become elevated **(3)** and they continue to circulate in the bloodstream until they are used for energy expenditure or are stored as fat. As the body is best equipped to manufacture long-chain saturated lipids, the triglycerides are ideal for storing as fat. It's hardly surprising then that the body, in response, puts on weight.

An elevated level of triglycerides is dangerous for several reasons: there is reason to believe that triglycerides work against HDL (high-density lipoprotein, the "good cholesterol"); also, they can attach themselves to the walls of blood vessels, adding to the risk factors if high blood pressure is already in the picture.

In this case, the triglycerides build upon the already narrowing vessel walls, and increase the risk for cardiovascular disease and stroke.

An interesting fact is that the fatty sheen on greasy skin is composed of triglycerides, so there might be a connection between a person having greasy skin and having a higher risk factor for adverse cardiac events due to elevated triglycerides.

WE WERE BORN WITH A SWEET TOOTH

Children tend to have more of a sweet tooth than adults. This dates back to our origins, when our chances of survival increased if we were lucky to feast on the sweet tasting (edible) as opposed to the bitter tasting (poisonous). Sweet tastes in nature are associated with non toxic and wholesome foods, and guarantee growth and energy essential to a developing brain. Naturally occurring sweetness found in fruits, berries, honey, milk, and breast milk doesn't give us any trouble; however, when sugar intake exceeds the 10 percent mark of our diet (established as an acceptable and healthy upper level) then problems arise.

CHILDREN AND SUGAR

A Finnish study showed that already between the ages 13 months to 9 years, the risk factors we know apply to cardiovascular disease are negatively impacted through sugar consumption (4). That study, known as STRIP, demonstrated that an increased intake of sugar was consistent with a higher intake of saturated long-chained fats, very little dietary fiber, and a large amount of cholesterol. The researchers found this to be evidence of an increased risk for cardiovascular disease, and it also showed that the overconsumption of sugar itself contributed to elevated blood lipids (as in triglycerides). Another interesting finding was that children who ate less sugar and more fiber than other children did not suffer a slower rate of growth, even though they consumed less calories overall.

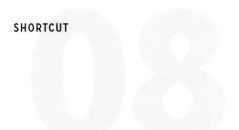

If the Label Says "Light" Leave It on the Shelf

"LIGHT" FOODS MAY MAKE YOU HEAVY

A few years back, I was invited to participate in a television program. The intent was to visit a grocery store and educate shoppers about healthy alternatives on the shelves. I was accompanied by a shopper who was seeking advice on how to improve her eating habits by making some simple changes to her grocery list. As we perused the different departments, I realized that her usual choices would definitely benefit from some tweaking. One of the changes I convinced her to make was to replace snack chips with nuts, and to buy flavored mineral water instead of soda.

We then hit the dairy aisle. She explained to me that she had learned to be very "sensible" and that she now chose to eat "light" yogurt with her breakfast cereal. She showed me the container where it was clearly marked that this was a "lighter" alternative.

My question is, lighter compared to what? A plain, original yogurt contains fewer calories than the light yogurt she usually picked. The reason is that the lighter version has a whopping sugar content of 13 percent, which is even more than what you'll find in a soda! That "light" food doesn't provide a nutritious breakfast—it's an item that's more suited to the candy aisle.

WE ARE BETTER INFORMED TODAY

The tide is turning in Sweden, and fewer products are now touted as "light," as the trend to replace fat with sugar is steadily losing ground. However, it's still a good habit to read labels carefully, as some light items in the dairy aisle now contain other dubious ingredients. Modified starch is sometimes used to add texture and firmness to a product; this is common practice among dairy manufacturers and is found in, among other things, "light" crème fraîche. And just because a product is not advertised as "light" doesn't mean that it is not filled with sweetener. Pasta sauce and many other ready-to-serve dishes are common examples of manufactured foods containing surprising amounts of sugar.

The trend toward "light" products is still very popular. Even though these people think they are doing well by eating healthier, but the "healthy" items they consume are still heavily sweetened.

ARE PRODUCTS LABELED "LIGHT" DANGEROUS?

There exist many conflicting opinions on the subject of "light" products; the critics who proffer the most scathing analysis of these diet foods usually highlight the various chemical artificial sweeteners used therein.

Aspartame, sucralose (Splenda), stevia, and erythritol are all extremely sweet tasting substances with little to no calorific value. I'll spend more time discussing these sweeteners in a later segment of the book, but I'll say now that according to current scientific evidence, the only one that has been negatively singled out is sucralose, even though, as with the other sugar alternatives listed above, it hasn't shown to be harmful when ingested. Saccharine, for its part, is the oldest artificial sweetener available on the market, but it's gradually being phased out as an ingredient and is being replaced by newer, better tasting alternatives.

Even if it is shown that artificial sweeteners are not actually harmful, it can nevertheless be said that there is nothing really healthy about them. As mentioned earlier, they can trigger sugar cravings in some people by increasing their ghrelin levels (see page 13). Others experience a cephalic response when tasting something sweet, that is, they have an insulin reaction. Yet another adverse side effect from artificial sweeteners is caused by their lack of carbohydrates: blood sugar levels tend to drop after you drink, for instance, a glass of light cola. When blood sugar is low, appetite and sugar cravings are stimulated, which is unfortunate if you are trying to avoid eating too many calories.

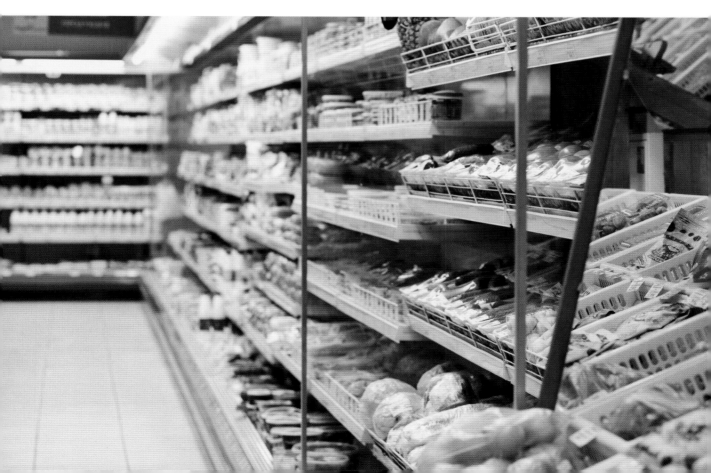

09

Foods with Added Sugar

SUGAR-LADEN ALTERNATIVES TO MILK

It's easy to become discouraged when you practice nutritional science. Over the last few years, many products have come on the market and have been promoted as healthy, when they, in fact, contain large amounts of sugar. Sugar is an inexpensive ingredient, so it's understandable that including it in certain foods is good for the manufacturer's profit margin. Nevertheless, it's highly unsuitable for your health.

One example of a food touted as "healthy" is soy milk. There are sugar-free versions of this product, but there are also many flavored kinds that contain added sugar, which make them far from ideal.

Once, after warning an audience about all the sugar added to soy milk, I received a complaint from an importer, who strongly maintained that there was no sugar added to the product.

A quick visit to the import company's website showed me that the information clearly stated that their milk product contained sugar. While there was a sugar-free alternative available, this was not the product the company was pushing. I often feel that it's a mad hatter's world out there when a product can be lauded for its health-giving properties even though it's full of sugar.

There are new products introduced constantly to replace cow's milk; hopefully in time and with heightened consumer awareness, these new substitutes will become healthier and far less sweetened.

Oat milk is another alternative food that has gained popularity, but even here you can't avoid finding varieties sweetened with sugar. To my despair, even delicious almond milk has been tampered with.

Rice milk is a product growing in popularity and I frequently see it in grocery stores that stock larger varieties of food. Yet, here again, I have only found the kind with added sugar.

As I've said before: it's important to read the labels carefully and check the ingredients, otherwise you might drink what amounts to a soda while believing it to be a healthy beverage.

OVER THE LAST FEW YEARS, MANY PRODUCTS HAVE COME ON THE MARKET AND BEEN PROMOTED AS HEALTHY, WHEN THEY, IN FACT, CONTAIN LARGE AMOUNTS OF SUGAR.

• •

WHEY BUTTER AND WHEY CHEESE

Swedish whey butter is another food product promoted as healthy. The manufacturer, Fjällbrynt, uses its website to reinforce this image by showing a cross-country skier in action, midway through a grueling workout.

If you are an avid exerciser, whey butter is not bad for you because it's highly caloric; the downside is that it contains sugar. The usual yellow whey butter is made up of about 5 percent sugar, while the light version has 4 percent. These levels are not alarmingly high, but it feels somehow misleading to market this product as outright healthy.

SUGAR IN WINE

Many of the world's wine-producing countries allow their wineries to add sugar to their product.

This process is called chaptalization, and was named after one of Napoleon's ministers of the interior—Jean-Antoine Chaptal—who encouraged this practice in order to help France unload a surplus of sugar beets.

Chaptalization raises the level of alcohol in wine, and in most cases all the added sugar is eaten up during fermentation and no traces of it remain in the finished product. If there is any leftover sugar, the winery must add sorbic acid to prevent the wine from fermenting further.

A laboratory test can easily tell which vintners add sugar, as the wine's sugar level will exceed 4 grams per liter (34 fluid ounces) and it will contain the aforementioned sorbic acid.

When I'm offered wine, I try to opt for one I know is free of added sugar. However, even in wines that contain some sugar, the amount is usually so minimal (around a fraction of an ounce per liter) that it causes virtually no ill effects to health. In fact it would take a vast amount of wine to reach unhealthy sugar levels—a quantity that would be unsound to drink, whether it were sugar-free or not.

10

Sugar in Our Restaurant Meals

IS SUGAR REALLY NECESSARY?

Have you ever taken a peek inside the kitchen of a Thai or Chinese restaurant? If so, you must have noticed sugar being added to the cooking pots. Sugar doesn't seem to faze populations throughout Asia, and this lack of concern might stem from the fact that malnutrition has historically been of greater concern than obesity in that part of the world.

I remember visiting a food fair in Cologne, Germany, and feeling awed while walking through the exhibition halls. Such an enormous space and such an incredible number of exhibitors! In the area devoted to beverages, I stopped at a Chinese stall where the vendor offered varieties of iced tea made from Chinese green tea. I sampled some and found them all very sweet, so I asked the seller if she had any sugar-free versions available, since the labels indicated that the ones I had tried contained lots of sugar. Her answer was a puzzled "whatever for?" She found it difficult to comprehend that anybody would prefer to drink unsweetened

iced tea, or any unsweetened beverage for that matter. She raised her eyebrows in astonishment at my request.

There is still very little marketing of sugar-free products in many areas throughout Asia, but there too, things are beginning to change. The Chinese, Thais, and other Asian people are now becoming increasingly aware of the dangers associated with excess sugar consumption.

SOUR MASKS SWEET

Sugar often heightens the taste of wok and curry recipes. Salty and sour dishes are finished off with a dash of sugar, and even in dishes heavy in oil and coconut milk, flavor is enhanced with a bit of sugar. Yet, it isn't necessary to add sugar to food. On Chinese and Thai menus, the unhealthiest dishes, excluding dessert, are those that emphasize the combination of sweet and sour.

The science of gustation tells us that sourness masks sweetness very effectively. Our taste buds will accept a higher grade

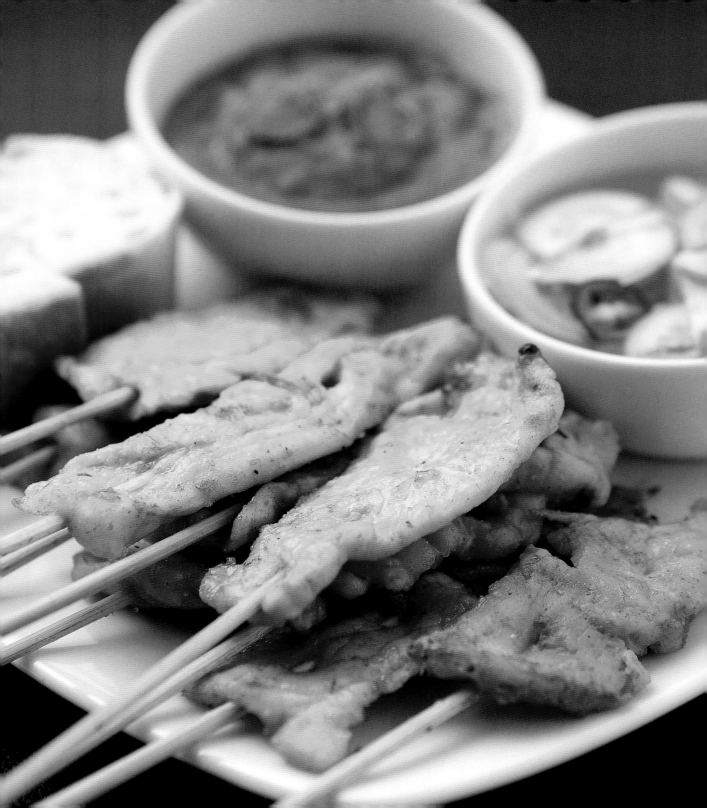

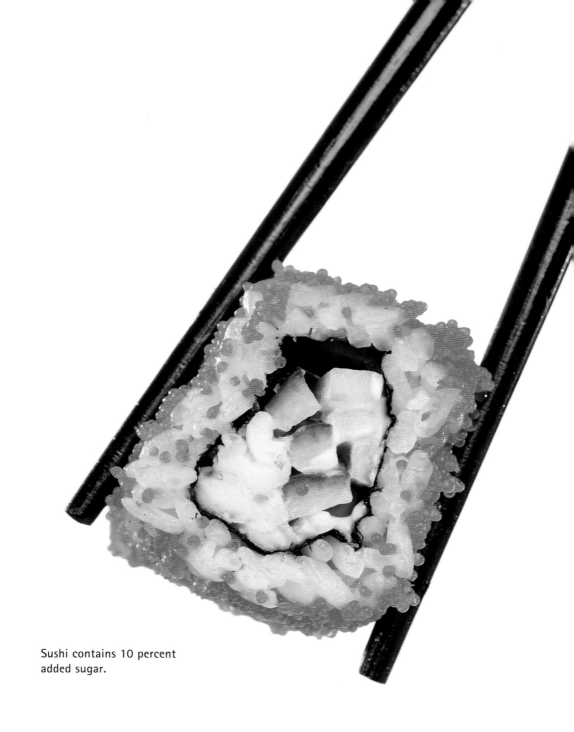

Sushi contains 10 percent
added sugar.

of sweetness if it is paired with acidity. You can perform a simple experiment to demonstrate this: leave a glass of carbonated sweetened soda in the refrigerator for several days until the carbonation has evaporated, then compare its taste with that of a freshly poured soda. The flat soda is nearly impossible to drink, as the sweetness has become overpowering. Carbonation is an acid and when it evaporates, the pH value of a beverage increases and the grade of sweetness intensifies. A sweet and sour dish without the balancing sourness would simply be too sweet and therefore off-putting.

Japanese cooking also considers sugar a critical ingredient. Teriyaki and Yakiniku come to mind, as the sugar content of those sauces makes them very sticky, more akin to fudge sauce than a savory sauce in consistency.

SUGAR-FREE SUSHI—DOES IT EXIST?

I cannot tell a lie: I love sushi. It's delicious, it's reasonably healthy, and is also extremely convenient to bring to lunch meetings or to order as takeout for dinner, if you're unable to enjoy it in a nice restaurant. It's often a good value too, and only someone with an allergy to fish or a committed vegan would have objections to such a meal. Most other people find something to like on a sushi menu. The wonderful salmon supplies a healthy dose of Omega-3 fat, vitamin D, and high protein content. Its pink color comes from a heart-healthy and fat-soluble pigment called astaxanthin, which is an antioxidant commonly found in a wide variety of fish and seafood.

The other ingredients found in a salmon sushi roll pose a problem, though: the rice is white rice, which is not as healthy as brown

OUR TASTE BUDS WILL ACCEPT A HIGHER GRADE OF SWEETNESS IF IT IS PAIRED WITH ACIDITY.

rice. The rice vinegar mixed into the rice is good; it slows down the glucose uptake, giving a simple piece of sushi the decent GI value of 70. But oh, the sugar, all that sugar! One piece of sushi contains more sugar than most of us would want to consume in a single day. What's interesting about this is that the sugar is totally unnecessary: use the right kind of rice and it will stick together and be easily pliable, and it's easy to wean yourself off the sugary taste.

OTHER RESTAURANT FARE

Even restaurants tend to add quite a lot of sugar to their dishes, but it isn't difficult to steer clear of the worst culprits. If a lunch dish comes with a side of jelly or jam, it's easy to simply leave it on the plate. Difficulties arise if you eat ready-made meals such as store-bought salsa, savory crêpes, meatballs, or meat sauce, as these dishes use sugar to both bring out their flavor, as well as to increase volume—all very inexpensively. If you are in doubt about a particular dish, you can ask the server for more information, as by law restaurant kitchens must state the ingredients they use in their offerings.

11

Stay Clear of Liquid Sugar

LIQUID SUGAR DOES NOT SATIATE

When you consume foods with added sugar, you experience a feeling of satiety, and you do get some nourishment from other ingredients. The problem with products that contain refined sugar in liquid form—sweetened beverages, for instance—is that they provide very little satiety. They only contribute excess calories, which are all too easy to consume in large quantities.

These include not only all sodas but fruit syrups, fruit drinks, energy drinks, sports drinks, and other sweetened beverages. Soups made from rosehip or blueberry, as well as fruit custards and puddings do provide a certain level of satiety due to their denser viscosity, but it doesn't make them healthier. They all contain unnecessary added sugar and there are better foods to enjoy as a snack or a treat.

DON'T COMPARE SODAS WITH JUICE

Occasionally, articles in the popular press will show that there is the same amount of sugar in a glass of fruit juice as there is in a glass of soda. This comparison is as irrelevant as saying that a glass of juice is equal to a glass of beer because they both contain the same amount of water.

Not all juices are created equally; fruit juices such as Sunny Delight and Kool-Aid have a lot of added sugars. Check the label when you buy juices. Make sure it contains 100 percent fruit juice and no other additives. Because the juice is un adulterated it provides vitamins, minerals, antioxidants, and even fiber (this is especially true if the juice contains fruit pulp), and not just a large amount of empty calories.

Many research studies have been made comparing juice with sodas. One notable example was a Japanese study of 27,585 men and women that found there was a direct correlation between soda consumption and type 2 diabetes. The strongest link was found among the women, where risk of developing diabetes doubled if soda was consumed daily (5).

This correlation was not found among the juice drinkers. Whether the beverage was

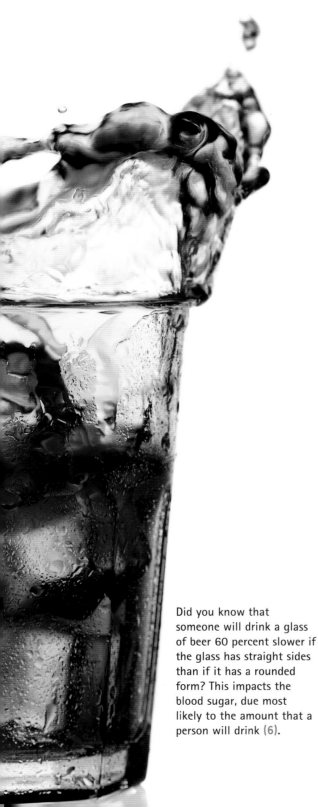

Did you know that someone will drink a glass of beer 60 percent slower if the glass has straight sides than if it has a rounded form? This impacts the blood sugar, due most likely to the amount that a person will drink **(6)**.

made from vegetables or fruit had no bearing on the findings. One theory on what causes type 2 diabetes is that free radicals damage the insulin receptors. As juice contains large amounts of free radical neutralizers, that is, antioxidants, the findings of the Japanese study support the theory. Another cause might be that soda's GI value is higher than juice, and high GI values are a well-known risk factor for diabetes.

FATTY LIVER

Fatty liver (or fatty liver disease) occurs when the liver is made up of more than 5 percent fat. Overweight individuals are more likely to suffer from it than people of normal weight, but fatty liver can still develop independently of body weight.

Excess consumption of sugar (especially refined fructose) and alcohol increase the risk of fatty liver, the reason being that the liver is reluctant to release large quantities of fructose and alcohol into the bloodstream, and instead will store it as fat. Fatty liver caused by being overweight is called nonalcoholic fatty liver disease, a condition that can be easily reversed if an individual loses weight.

It's important to stay within a normal weight range in order to keep insulin sensitivity intact, as the liver will not accept a lot of blood sugar if it is saturated with fat. It will run out of storage space and will no longer be receptive to insulin, and a liver that becomes insulin resistant is at the preliminary stage of type 2 diabetes.

In about 10 percent of those who suffer from a fatty liver, the condition can lead to inflammation, which itself can turn into cirrhosis of the liver, or liver cancer. Therefore, fatty liver must be treated as a very serious affliction.

Excessive soda consumption puts the liver at risk. Several studies have shown a strong correlation between fatty liver and soda consumption (7,8,9). One study showed, for example, that 80 percent of subjects diagnosed with fatty liver consumed ½ liter (17 fluid ounces) of soda a day, while only 17 percent of the healthy subjects drank a comparable amount (8).

PANCREATIC CANCER

Pancreatic cancer is considered a very serious ailment due to having one of the poorest survival prognoses of all cancers. Soda, with its large amount of sugar and simple carbohydrates, provides a huge glucose load and more than likely overburdens the pancreas. The pancreas produces the hormone insulin, and secretes it into the bloodstream where the body needs it to keep the blood sugar balanced. There are several studies, which when taken into account concurrently, show an alarming connection: the risk factor for developing pancreatic cancer becomes frighteningly real with soda drinking (10).

Here again we need to take care to avoid comparing soda to juice: a large study involving more than 60,000 test subjects showed that there was a clear correlation between soda consumption and pancreatic cancer, but failed to show a similar correlation with juice consumption (11).

PREMATURE BIRTH

Many women drink soda, both sweetened with sugar and sweetened with artificial sweeteners, during their pregnancy. They should be aware that this habit is not without risks. The more soda they consume, the more they run the risk of giving birth prematurely (12).

This holds true whether they drink artificially sweetened soda and sugar-sweetened soda, so the problem isn't from the ingestion of sugar itself.

Perhaps it's the caffeine in the sodas that's the real culprit? What about its acidity? Whatever the case may be, it's clear it isn't healthy to consume excessive amounts of sugar during pregnancy. By now you've come to understand

SODA AND OBESITY

Very few food items are as fattening, as well as non filling, as soda, with its large amount of liquid empty calories. Many studies show soda to be the most fattening item consumed by both children and adults (19, 20, 21). To make matters worse, it seems as though people with a genetic predisposition for being overweight are also most likely to be drawn to soda (22). Replacing classic soda with light soda seems to alleviate the problem of weight gain (23), even though it might bring on other health issues.

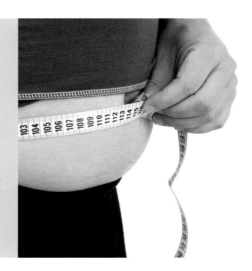

that sugar impacts health in a myriad of negative ways; add to these the risk of putting on too much pregnancy weight if sugar consumption gets out of hand.

CARDIOVASCULAR DISEASE

It's hardly surprising to learn that soda consumption increases the risk for cardiovascular disease, now that you know the large glucose load it provides. In a large study where 42,883 participating male subjects were followed over a period of 22 years, it became apparent that the one fifth of the participants who drank the largest amount of soda also had a 20 percent higher risk of developing cardiovascular disease (13). Soda consumption, as expected, heightened several risk factors, such as elevated blood lipids, C-reactive protein, and lowered HDL (the good cholesterol). However, the artificially sweetened "light" soda did not produce increased risk factors.

HIGH BLOOD PRESSURE

Drinking soda daily elevates blood pressure (14). This in turn is a serious risk factor for stroke, and in time can also lead to cardiovascular disease. It's not exactly clear what causes the elevated blood pressure, but it is believed that insulin may play a part. It's interesting to note that even artificially sweetened sodas have this effect, which means something other than sweeteners is involved. Perhaps the sodas somehow alter the mineral balance; carbonation has been mentioned as a possible culprit. Phosphoric acid found in colas might also be considered suspect.

COCA-COLA, COULD IT GET ANY WORSE?

Coca-Cola was invented in Atlanta, GA, in 1886 by a chemist named John Pemberton.

He mixed carbonated water, phosphoric acid, caffeine, sugar, sugar-derived colorant, and flavorings. Today, this mixture is known as the most popular soda in the world.

Millions of people drink Coca-Cola every day, so it deserves a closer look. I don't believe that a glass or two per week is going to do you any harm; the problem is that it contains caffeine, which can be addictive, and thus it is not uncommon for children and teenagers as well as adults to consume large quantities of it daily.

Apart from health problems brought on by sugar, we also know that cola drinks increase the risk for osteoporosis because the phosphoric acid binds to calcium, and because cola often replaces milk as the primary beverage with meals (15).

Icelandic research has shown that if someone drinks cola three or more times per week, he or she runs a tripled risk for tooth enamel erosion (16).

Phosphoric acid even seems to inflict damage on the kidneys, and the increased risk for kidney disease is present whether you drink the light or sugar-sweetened original cola (17).

A study using rats also showed that animals that were given Coca-Cola instead of water to drink in their cages suffered higher instances of different forms of cancer (18). Even though these studies involved animals and not human subjects, they still give cause for alarm, as the effects of the daily cola drink on the rats were so pronounced. It would be highly unethical to replicate this kind of study using human participants, but perhaps some future study will look into possible links between cola consumption in humans and cancer.

12

How to Prevent a Sugar Slump

SUGAR SLUMPS LESSEN QUALITY OF LIFE

I'm sure you've experienced a sugar slump—also called crash—at least once. That feeling of drowsiness is the drugged out–like state induced by eating sweets and simple carbohydrates. The most common illustration of this phenomenon is when people get the irresistible urge to take a nap after a big feast such as Thanksgiving dinner. Both the amount of food and the rate of absorption of the carbohydrates affects whether you feel drowsy or not. If you tend to feel sleepy in the afternoon, it's more than likely you are feeling the effects of a sugar slump.

There are ways to lessen this problem: Avoid refined sugar completely, eat fewer carbohydrates, and only eat carbohydrates with low GI value. Experiencing sugar crashes regularly is unhealthy, and can be a sign of impeding diabetes. Many who are diagnosed with diabetes also feel drowsy after mealtimes, so take heed. However, if it only occurs on rare occasions when you eat too much or too many of the wrong foods, it's a perfectly natural and temporary reaction.

WHAT HAPPENS IN THE BODY DURING A SUGAR SLUMP?

What happens in the body during a sugar crash makes for a fascinating physiological story. There is a balance in the blood between different amino acids. You get the essential amino acids from the proteins you eat, which are of utmost importance because they're necessary to generate new proteins such as muscles and body tissues. Others, however, are used as building blocks for the brain's different neurotransmitters. Whichever amino acids are present in the blood will affect this process.

There is a kind of teamwork that takes place between the branched chain amino acides leucine, isoleucine, and valine, as well as the amino acid tryptophan. These essential acids share the same transport mechanism to the brain. The branched chain amino acids move into the muscles and are used as building blocks when the body releases insulin, which happens when you eat carbohydrates. The simpler the carbohydrates and the more of them you eat, the more insulin is released into the bloodstream, which in turn decreases the levels of leucine, isoleucine, and valine in the blood. As a result, the balance of tryptophan and the grenade amino acids shifts so that more tryptophan enters the brain. As serotonin production correlates directly to the level of tryptophan, this brings on a feeling of relaxation, pleasure, and satiety, but also of sluggishness.

This can create a problem because it leads to inactivity (and perhaps a nap), which in turn sends the level of blood sugar spiking. When you're asleep, your muscles are inactive and don't use up any glucose, which leads to increased and unhealthy blood sugar levels.

IF YOU HAVE EATEN TOO MUCH

If you've eaten a copious lunch and feel drowsy afterward, there are things you can do to counteract the undesirable effect:

● Drink a big glass of water to dilute the contents of your stomach, which will slow down the release of sugar in the bloodstream.
● Drink a cup of tea or coffee with a dash of ground cinnamon in it. Both the drink and the cinnamon will keep the blood sugar level, and the caffeine will make you feel more alert.
● Take a brisk walk, or engage in some form of exercise for at least 30 minutes. It would be even better if you can make it last 1 hour. That way you will increase your muscles' use of glucose, decrease the level of insulin, and the blood chemistry can start normalizing.

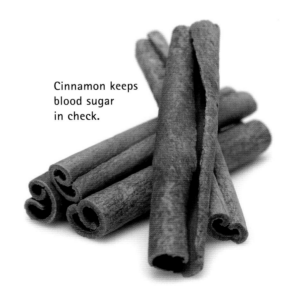

Cinnamon keeps blood sugar in check.

13

Use Raw Cane Sugar Instead of Refined Sugar

THE WORLD'S MOST CULTIVATED CROP

Sugarcane is the world's largest cultivated crop, one of the main reasons being that it is used to make ethanol.

But, first and foremost, sugarcane is used to manufacture sugar for human consumption; 1.7 billion tons of sugar is produced each year (2010), in more than 90 countries, including Brazil, its biggest manufacturer.

HEALTHIER THAN REFINED SUGAR

Raw cane sugar is the unrefined version of cane sugar, but does this imply that it's healthier than refined sugar?

Raw cane sugar is derived from sugarcane in the form of evaporated juice. This means that apart from the sucrose, the juice retains all its other nutrients, including vitamins, minerals, antioxidants, and quite a lot of other natural elements. While antioxidants aren't plentiful, raw cane sugar still contains 0.1 mmol per 100 grams (3.5 ounces), compared to refined sugar that in general contains no antioxidants whatsoever.

Other sugars such as maple syrup, brown (muscovado) sugar, and honey have between 0.2 and 0.7 mmol antioxidants per 100 gram (3.5 ounces).

RAW CANE SUGAR STIMULATES THE IMMUNE SYSTEM

FRAP (Fluorescence Recovery After Photobleaching) and ORAC (Oxygen Radical Absorbance Capacity) are two methods used to measure antioxidant content. If, hypothetically, we were to replace all sugar in an average diet with raw cane sugar, we would be talking about something in the range of 130 grams (4.5 ounces) a day; the antioxidant content would be equal to that of a portion of fruit or nuts [24]. In animal studies, raw cane sugar has proven to stimulate the immune system [25] and even to protect against Röntgen radiation [26].

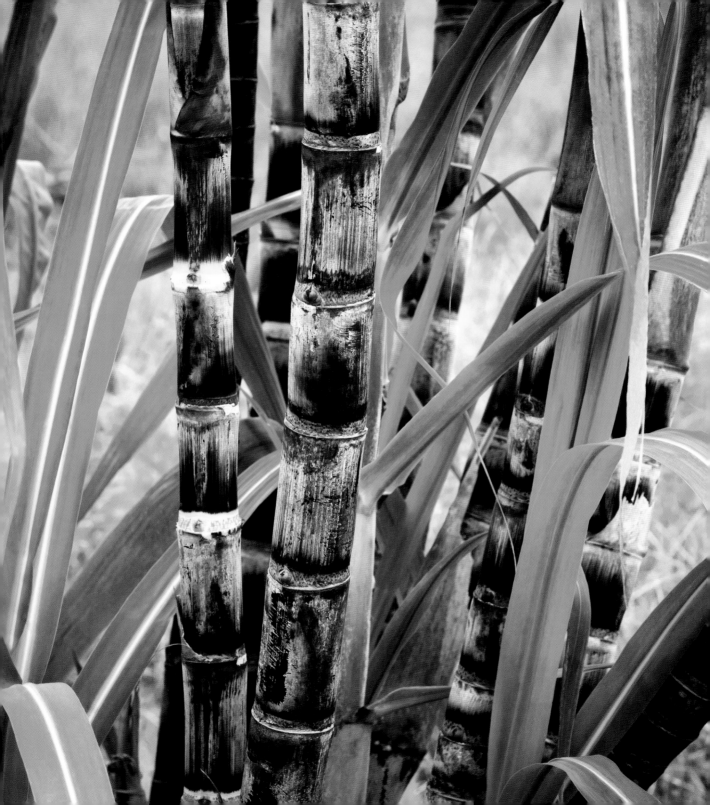

CONTRIBUTING TO REDUCED GI

Theoretically, raw cane sugar could have a lower GI value than refined sugar, but more importantly, it could lower the GI value of starchy foods when consumed in tandem.

This is because raw cane sugar contains a bioflavonoid that inhibits the enzymes responsible for breaking down starches. As a result, raw cane sugar would probably lower the GI value of, say, a cinnamon roll, or some other starch-heavy food.

If we give test subjects around 15 milligrams of this bioflavonoid (the amount found in a reasonable amount of raw cane sugar), the GI value-lowering effect would reach 37 percent **(27)**.

Raw cane sugar also contains some palatinose (isomaltulose), sugar that contributes to giving it a lower GI value.

Palatinose is a sugar with a chemical make up that's very similar to sucrose, as it's part fructose and part glucose. The difference lies in how the molecules bind: in palatinose the connection breaks down at a much slower rate than in sucrose; consequently, the sugars enter the bloodstream at a more moderate pace.

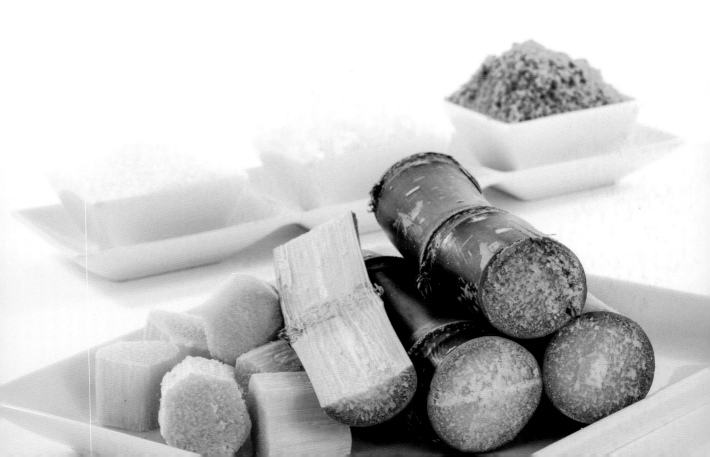

14

Coconut—It's All Good

COCONUT SUGAR

I had never encountered coconut sugar until I took a culinary trip to Thailand.

We traveled to Hua Hin to cook alongside a highly esteemed chef. While I was excited by this unique opportunity, I became worried when he mentioned that some dishes—mango salad with shrimp, and a red curry chicken dish—had sugar among the ingredients.

My concerns vanished, however, as soon as I saw what he meant by the word "sugar." He used coconut sugar, which is brown and has a delicious, rich flavor. Without really knowing anything more about this sweetener, I accepted it as part of the recipes. The amounts used were so small, it could be considered fairly benign; furthermore the brown color meant that the sugar contained some antioxidants.

Upon my return home, I read up on this ingredient and was delighted to find that coconut sugar is a good choice if you need to sweeten a dish, as it contains several important nutrients and the GI value is only 35.

Compared to raw cane sugar's GI value of 50 and refined sugar's GI value of 80, this is a vast improvement.

Coconut sugar is derived from the nectar of the coconut palm flower, and is naturally rich in nutrients such as magnesium, potassium, iron, and zinc. It also contains a healthy dose of vitamin B1, B2, B3, and B6. Coconut sugar is also called palm sugar, but be careful: some palm sugar is derived from the date palm. As coconut sugar is just as sweet as refined sugar, it can be used in lieu of refined sugar in the exact same quantities, ounce for ounce.

XYLOSE IN COCONUT SHELLS

The hard brown coconut shell, which is not edible in its raw form, contains the sugar xylose, also called wood sugar. Xylose is not the same as coconut sugar but has shown great promise in regulating blood sugar, so I want to mention it here.

In the medical field, xylose is used to detect malabsorption of nutrients and is considered safe for consumption. Of interest is that xylose not only slows the breakdown of starches but also of sucrose, which produces a longer blood glucose curve **(28)**. Naturally this leads to lower insulin release.

Perhaps xylose is tomorrow's ingredient for staples like breads, baked goods, and breakfast cereals. It might even become the key to healthier foods for diabetics and everybody who needs to keep their blood sugar under control.

FAT AND PROTEIN IN COCONUTS

Coconut fat is good for us. We know this now after many years' study. Comprised of 60 to 70 percent short- and medium-chain fatty acids, this saturated fat—very little of which is stored and is easily used for energy—is an excellent fat to eat. It slows down absorption of sugar, thereby contributing to a better blood sugar curve. Coconut fat also provides blood sugar control, improved stamina, and general good health.

The coconut's protein is very rich in the amino acid arginine, which in nutritional physiology is classified as a "nitrogen donor." Arginine expands blood vessels and has shown, when used in studies of diabetic animals, to aid in the repair of beta cells **(29)**. As these are the insulin-producing cells in the pancreas, this fantastic characteristic could, in theory, wipe out type 1 diabetes, even in humans. Future research will show whether that's the case, but until then we can eat coconuts to our heart's content. Keep in mind, too, that most of the protein is contained in the white, firm coconut meat, which can be bought fresh or grated.

COCONUT WATER IMPROVES BLOOD SUGAR

We know today that the meat, fat, and shell from coconuts aid blood sugar control through different ways. But even coconut water has the potential to balance blood sugar. This water comes from the young, green coconut, and is known in many tropical countries as a true thirst-quencher. It contains high levels of potassium as well as many antioxidants and other nutrients beneficial for your health.

So far, studies on coconut water have been limited to animal studies, but the results look promising: the animals were shown to have been protected against oxidative stress—the damage caused by free radicals—and also to have seen improvement to their insulin sensitivity **(30, 31)**. As coconut water is common in stores today, why not try it next time you're looking for a refreshing drink?

COCONUT WATER IS KNOWN AS A GOOD WAY TO HYDRATE BECAUSE OF ITS ELECTROLYTE CONTENT.

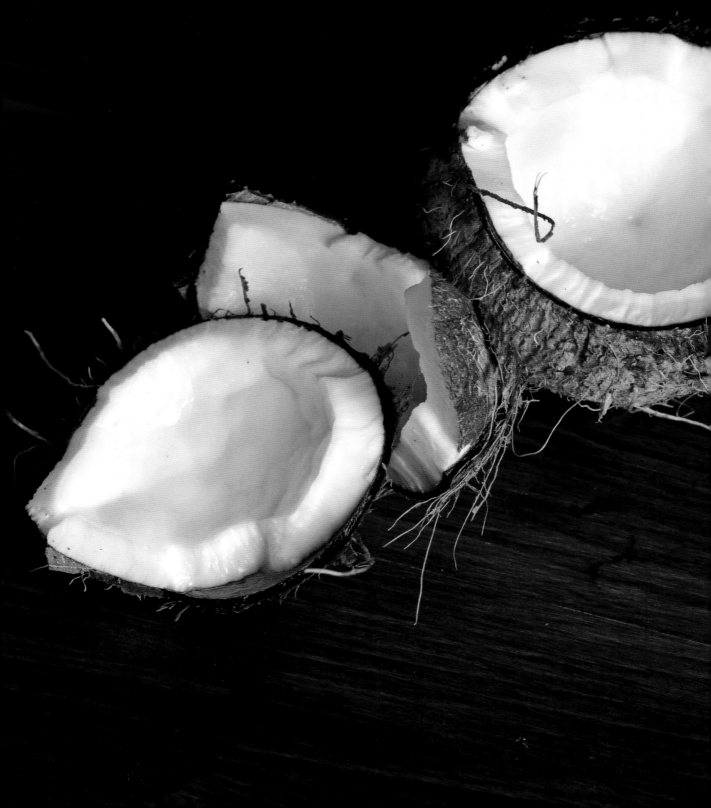

15

Choose the Right Sweetener

SUCRALOSE—THE WORST ALTERNATIVE

When sucralose was launched in Europe in 2004, many believed it to be the perfect artificial sweetener. Sucralose is chemically very similar to sucrose, but has a sweetening power 500 to 600 times greater than sugar, which renders Sucralose virtually non caloric. It is manufactured through the chlorination of sucrose, it is very heat-stable, and can be used in combination with acidic or neutral-tasting ingredients.

Other well-known chlorinated organic compounds are DDT (dichlorodiphenyltri-chloroethane) and PCB (polychlorinated biphenyl), both of which have a long decomposition time, which in turn makes them environmentally hazardous. The same extended decomposition rate applies to sucra-lose, which makes it baffling that a consensus has not yet been reached as to whether the substance is dangerous to eat. Sucralose travels through water purification plants without deteriorating, and we still don't know the full range of its effects on a wide variety of fauna and flora in lakes and rivers. We are aware that DDT and PCB are hazardous materials due in part to their long half-life, so perhaps we will end up classifying sucralose as dangerous sometime in the future.

Sucralose residue has been proven to have a negative effect on marine life. A Swedish study showed that the water flea, Daphnia magna, is affected by sucralose through its increased rate of motion in the water, as well as in its tendency to swim nearer to the surface (32). The same study also showed that gammarids took longer to find food and seek shelter in water tainted by sucralose.

ASPARTAME—NOT DESERVING OF ITS BAD REPUTATION

Aspartame is an artificial sweetener consisting of L-aspartic acid and L-phenylala-nine, two amino acids naturally found in our foods. Aspartame is about 200 times sweeter than sucrose and is considered non caloric. Since its approval in the United States in 1974,

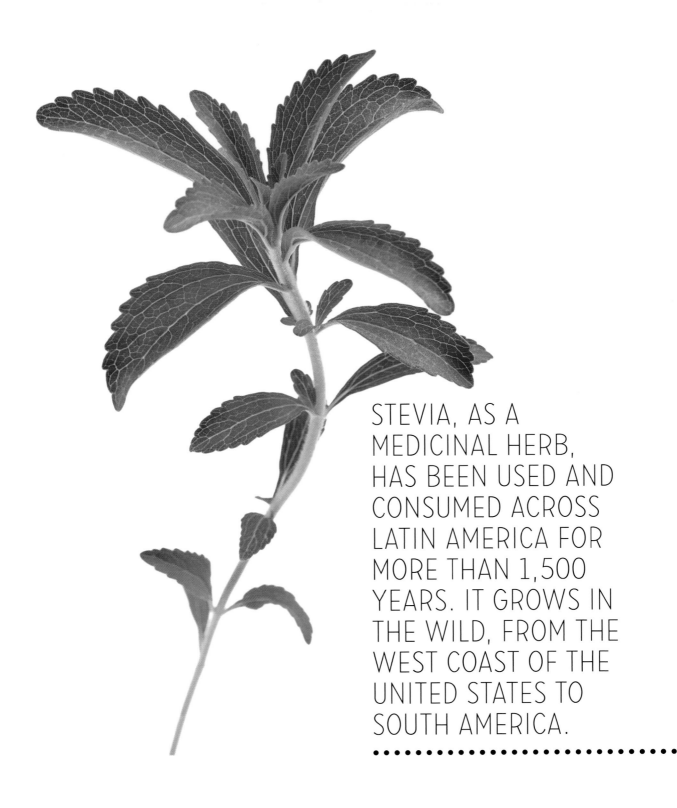

STEVIA, AS A MEDICINAL HERB, HAS BEEN USED AND CONSUMED ACROSS LATIN AMERICA FOR MORE THAN 1,500 YEARS. IT GROWS IN THE WILD, FROM THE WEST COAST OF THE UNITED STATES TO SOUTH AMERICA.

it has come under plenty of scrutiny and criticism, the latter without much foundation.

One thing that fuels criticism is that products sweetened with aspartame carry the warning "contains L-phenylalanine," which has been misconstrued by some to mean that it's dangerous to ingest. There is L-phenylalanine in nearly all foods, but only people suffering from a specific genetic metabolic disease called phenylketonuria need to be cautious. They have a severely diminished ability to metabolize L-phenylalanine and eating too much of it can sicken them, so it's important that they be wary of products containing L-phenylalanine. For 99.9 percent of the population who don't suffer from this genetic trait, however, the presence or absence of L-phenylalanine in their food carries no significance.

Another reason the naysayers worry about aspartame is that its breakdown produces methanol. This alcohol is feared because when it's added to heighten the alcoholic content of homemade liquor, it has been known to cause poisoning, blindness, even death. The methanol produced by normal soda consumption is so small that the body has time to get rid of it through the normal processes of digestion long before it can do any harm. There is actually more naturally occurring

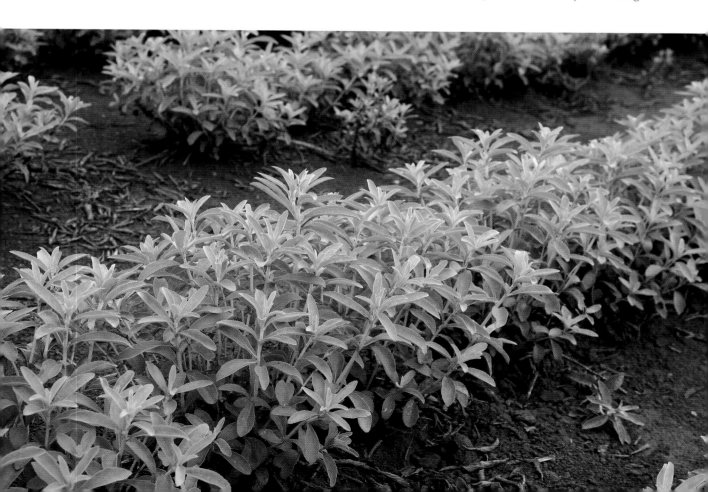

methanol in grapefruit juice than what can be found in a glass of diet soda.

Aspartame as an artificial sweetener is approved for use in more than 90 countries, so I feel it is perfectly fine to replace sugar with reasonable amounts of aspartame. That said, it's not nutritious in any way, and can increase cravings for sweet things; it may even cause an insulin response in sensitive people. For that reason, it is better to avoid it if possible.

STEVIA—THE FASHIONABLE SWEETENER

The latest sweetener approved by the EU (European Union) is stevia, but it has a long history of use elsewhere.

Stevia, Stevia rebeudiana, a medicinal herb, has been used and consumed across Latin America for more than 1,500 years. It grows wild from the West Coast of the United States to South America, and is cultivated in many Asian countries. China is the world's leading producer of stevia.

The stevia flavor is slower to blossom, and it lingers longer than sucrose; some extracts have a hint of licorice, and sometimes even a slight bitter aftertaste. The sweetness is produced by steviol glycosides (stevioside and rebaudioside), and is up to 300 times sweeter than sucrose. This means that very little goes a long way. Stevia is heat stable, and since it can be used in conjunction with acids it is suitable for use in sodas and fruit syrups. Coca-Cola uses stevia in certain markets—Japan, for one. Aspartame is not approved for use in Japan, which has given stevia a competitive advantage since its introduction at the beginning of the 1970s; today its market share is approximately 40 percent. For that reason, much research on stevia has taken place in Japan,

and the results, along with forty years of incorporating stevia in food to no ill effect, have shown that stevia is both safe and healthy to use as a sweetener **(33)**.

Chemically, stevia is made up of glucose and aglycone. The glucose contributes sweetness, but due to the infinitesimal amount of stevia needed, it doesn't impact blood glucose in any measurable way. This makes stevia safe for diabetics, and many food scientists feel that stevia is a superior sweetener, due to both the nature of its sugars and as a non caloric choice for diabetics **(34)**. Research shows that stevia provokes less insulin response than both aspartame and, naturally, sucrose **(35)**.

Erythritol, a sugar alcohol, was discovered as early as 1848; it exists naturally in fruits such as pears and melons, as well as in certain fungi and in many fermented products. At first glance, there are many positive aspects to erythritol: first, it looks and tastes like sucrose. It already has natural bulk, so it's not necessary to add a bulking agent to bind the sweetening agent in foods. It is very suitable for food preparation and baking. Second, erythritol does not have the same laxative or gassy side effects of many other sugar alcohols. This means you don't have to limit your intake for fear that your stomach will balloon, as might be the case after eating something containing maltitol or xylitol. The reason is that 90 percent of erythritol is broken down in the small intestine, so it never reaches the large intestine where it would, with aid of bacteria, ferment and cause gastric distress. The erythritol that is absorbed is eliminated in the urine more or less intact. It has 0.24 calories per gram, but is not actually metabolized and so is considered nutritionally non caloric.

16

Focus on the Real Culprits

DON'T STRAIN GNATS BUT SWALLOW CAMELS

Having my own line of foods affords me the opportunity to visit grocery stores all over Sweden. It's a great way to meet consumers, and people often approach me to talk about their eating habits. Sometimes I feel that they're looking for some sort of reassurance that they're on the right path, and it's perhaps not surprising that many who want to share their story or seek out further information already have pretty good diets.

I remember meeting a very nice woman in her forties who was already pretty knowledgeable about how to eat healthy. She pointed to the sugar-free sliced ham in her shopping cart: the package stated that it contained "no added sugar," and upon checking the ingredients list I found no sugar, no syrup, or any other ingredient to sweeten or bulk up the product to increase its manufacturer's profit margin.

"Surely this is much healthier than the usual sliced ham," she said, and I agreed. However, before I had time to explain that the tiny amount of sugar in a slice of deli ham hardly made any difference when part of a reasonable diet, she had already thanked me and was back to perusing the aisles. When I saw her next, she was helping herself to an assortment of favorite sweets from the candy bins.

I had to smile to myself. It fascinates me that she could put so much energy into finding an item that would decrease her daily sugar intake by a few paltry grains, and then happily fill up on candy, which is made of little else but sugar, and worse yet, is full of chemical additives.

Strain out gnats but swallow camels was a very fitting expression for this sort of conundrum.

PICK YOUR BATTLES

This doesn't mean you shouldn't strive to find non sugar alternatives, but there needs to be a clear health benefit to make your effort worthwhile.

The nice woman in the grocery store would have had to consume the entire package of

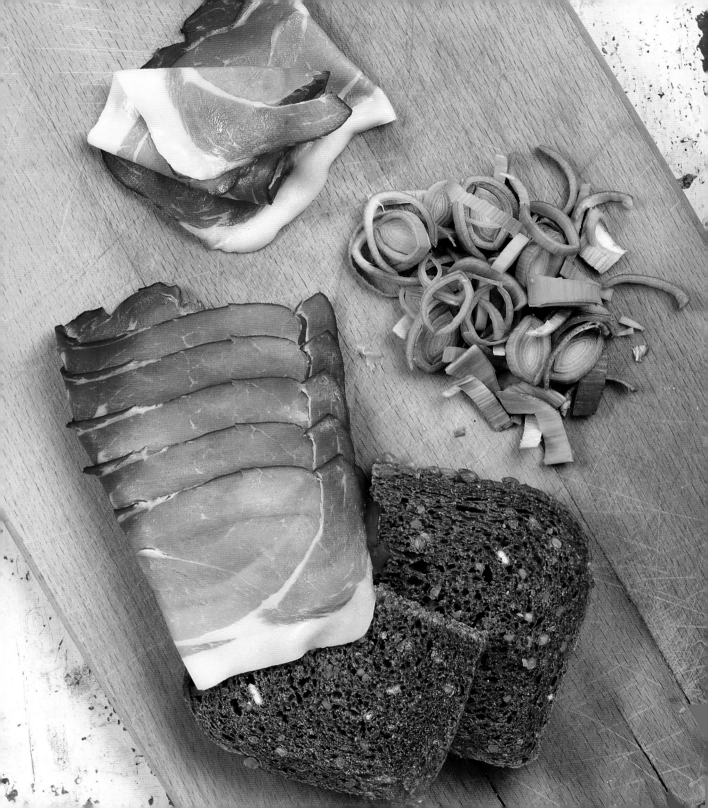

sugar-cured ham slices to ingest anywhere near the amount of sugar of one of those pieces of candy. The ham also provided her with some sound nutrition, which would have counteracted the negative effects of sugar.

Brined and sugar-cured chicken is another example of a food item with a relatively low sugar level, but that still causes some degree of anxiety among health-conscious consumers. Of course the best option is to pick a sugar-free alternative for your meal, but it's hardly the end of the world if you occasionally indulge in a piece of frozen chicken breast that contains a small amount of glucose preservative.

What's important is to choose sugar-free alternatives for the foods you eat habitually, or on a daily basis. Cook from scratch, use fresh produce, and don't add sugar to your dishes. If you feel tired, take a nap instead of finding your pick-me-up in a piece of chocolate. If you are unable to rest for a little while, perhaps drinking a cup of coffee will energize you. It's keeping a close eye on, and limiting, everyday, thoughtless sugar consumption that makes for good health.

SUGAR IN THE SCHOOLS

Many parents are unhappy about the amount of sugary foods still being served in our schools' and pre schools' cafeterias. It's true that added sugar lurks in the apple compôte, the sweetened yogurt, and the whey butter. However, as long as our children also eat wholesome and nutritious meals at home, they shouldn't reach anywhere near the 5 percent of daily calories from sugar that WHO has deemed to be the acceptable upper limit.

I do recommend that all parents stay involved and informed about the daily menu options of their kids' pre school and/ or school cafeterias. If they serve sweetened fruit soup each week, for example, this might be something to consider modifying; it's also good to limit sugar intake between meals. Most important, however, is to find the right balance, because if you're too stringent or restrictive of your kids' sugar intake, and by extension their food consumption, you run the risk of them not getting enough nourishment to foster proper growth, concentration, and stamina.

I DO RECOMMEND THAT PARENTS STAY INVOLVED AND INFORMED ABOUT THE DAILY MENU OFFERINGS IN PRE-SCHOOL AND SCHOOL CAFETERIAS. IT IS IMPORTANT TO LIMIT SUGAR BETWEEN MEALS.

17

Break the Sugar Addiction

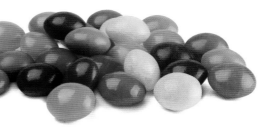

ARE YOU ADDICTED TO SUGAR?

It's common to compare sugar to narcotics, but is it really that addicting?

Below is a list of behaviors associated with addiction, prepared to fit sugar addiction. Do any of these apply to you?

● Your emphasis on sugar is affecting your daily life in a negative way.

● You feel as though you have no control over your sugar intake.

● You are aware that you eat too much sugar.

● You need more and more sugar to achieve the desired effect.

● You feel a psychological dependency on sugar, which varies in strength from weak to very strong, as in: "I could kill for some candy."

● You experience withdrawal symptoms after a few days without sugar in the form of headaches, mood swings, shakiness, anxiety, restlessness, and sleeplessness.

● You feel that you need to eat sugar, or you'll compensate by acting out in destructive ways, for example, shopping sprees, excess gambling, practicing unsafe sex, or behaving in other unproductive ways to lessen the withdrawal symptoms.

● You suffer negative consequences, either in yourself or in your surroundings, due to excessive sugar consumption. Perhaps in the form of incidents at work or at home, or you find that you are no longer as active in former healthy interests and pursuits.

● You keep consuming more sugar, and it happens more often than you mean it to.

● You continue to consume large quantities of sugar even though you are aware that it's detrimental to your health.

A REASONABLE THEORY

The theory that sugar is as addictive as hard drugs is reasonable, because sugar promotes the release of endorphins, which bind to the same receptors as heroin, those we call the "opiate receptors." Endorphins are often described as "the body's own morphine"—heroin's chemical relative. While it's erroneous to equate the two phenomena of drug addiction and sugar dependency, since heroin's effect is far more intense and its addiction a lot more difficult to break, there are some similarities. Both sugar and heroin are calming and dull anxiety, which could hold a strong attraction for someone troubled or depressed.

Sugar's morphine-like effect seems to be stronger on children than adults. During a routine visit to an ophthalmologist, my son (who was then around six months old) was far from cooperative. He screamed bloody murder and he wouldn't open his eyes; he punched, hit, and kicked until the nurse brought out her "magic potion," a pipette filled with a syrupy solution. She administered a few drops into my son's mouth, and the effect was immediate: he relaxed completely. The examination then proceeded without any further problems, but it was both frightening and fascinating to witness sugar's power over my son.

RESEARCH ON SUGAR ADDICTION

A study published in 1987 showed sugar's effect on pain relief, and that this effect could be blocked by a pharmaceutical agent that is also commonly used to counteract the effect of morphine **(36)**. In 1997, Kathleen DesMaisons stated in her book, *Potatoes Not Prozac* that sugar addiction is a term that is scientifically viable, as she could indeed show that it corresponds to the definition found in the DSM-IV (*Diagnostic and Statistical Manual of Mental Disorders*, Fourth Edition). This is the official diagnostic system for mental disorders used by the medical profession in the United States, so this lends a certain weight to her statement. Further clinical research supports the theory of the existence of sugar addiction: A study conducted in 2008 showed that eating sugar increased the level of opiates and dopamine in the brain, the substances that produce a feeling of calm and of reward **(37)**. Nobody questions the fact that drugs operating by the very same mechanisms are highly addictive. A newer study, dated 2012, demonstrated that someone who frequently consumes ice cream then often feels less satisfied by drinking a milkshake **(38)**. By using an MRI scanner it was possible to see exactly how the brain was stimulated by different stimuli, and how a person more accustomed to ice cream might get less "reward" from a milkshake. This phenomenon is called habituation, and it can be observed with other drugs—offering hard evidence that sugar addiction is real.

REAL-LIFE CASES

Throughout my career, I have met individuals with serious sugar addiction who display behavior patterns similar to those of heroin addicts. The big difference being that the former usually don't have to turn to crime to support their habit.

Let me offer you an example: I was a panelist on the Swedish television program, *Toppform* (*Top Fitness*), where I was the nutrition expert. One of the participants was a young woman in her twenties who ate far too much candy and who had turned to the show for help. I had no idea how many sweets she consumed until I interviewed her and she gave me the details. Upon waking, she would reach down and retrieve a Snickers Bar from a stash she kept under her bed, and eat it before even setting her feet on the floor. Her breakfast consisted of light yogurt covered with frosted flakes.

At lunch she ate very little, but she did drink soda. She also kept nibbling throughout the day, but since she worked at a candy store(!), her snacks were hardly of the health-conscious nuts-and-seeds variety. More often than not, her evening meal consisted of takeout food, with soda, which was then followed by a dessert of soft-serve ice cream. It probably goes without saying that this young woman had elevated lipid levels and was overweight, even though she was still young.

I calculated that 60 to 70 percent of her calories came from sugar, and I wouldn't hesitate to call her a sugar addict. Her addiction would in all likelihood shorten her life span if she didn't modify her eating patterns drastically.

HOW DO YOU FREE YOURSELF FROM SUGAR ADDICTION?

There are several methods to fight sugar addiction. First, start exercising. Exercise and physical activity are possibly the most effective method out there, and you can read more about it on page 82.

Second, never consciously put anything sweet in your mouth. Avoid all diet or "lite/light" products, and anything with added sugar. If you are truly addicted to sugar, it's possible that your craving will rear its head at even the faintest taste of sweetness—from fruits and berries, for instance—the way in which an alcoholic might fall off the wagon after eating a rum-flavored truffle. You'll have to work at reducing your body's ghrelin levels by abstaining from sweets, and derive feelings of reward from other channels, many of which can be found through exercise and workout programs.

Third, it of utmost importance to keep your blood glucose stable by eating meals at regular intervals throughout the day, as dips in blood sugar will make you hungry and might rev up your craving for sweets.

A good way to handle this is to eat carbohydrates with low GI value; removing all carbohydrates might counteract your efforts by triggering cravings for sweets.

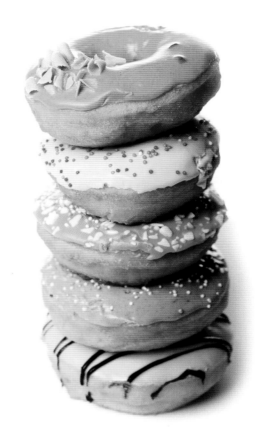

SUGAR CONSUMPTION INCREASES OPIATES AND DOPAMINE LEVELS IN THE BRAIN, PRODUCING FEELINGS OF CALM AND REWARD.

18

Sugar and Cancer

A PROVEN CORRELATION WITH CANCER

Do you believe that artificial sweeteners are carcinogenic, and that sucrose is natural and therefore safer to eat? If so, you have another thing coming! There is no substantiated research that shows a link between artificial sweeteners and cancer in humans, while there is much that shows a correlation between sugar and different types of cancer.

There are several explanations as to why sugar increases the risk for cancer. One is that sugar releases insulin and IGF-1 (insulin-like growth factor-1), both hormones known to speed up cell division. When this occurs, there is an increased risk of DNA damage, which, if it does not repair itself, will instead cause a mutation, which could eventually turn into cancer.

Another possible reason is that you need vitamin B in order to metabolize carbohydrates, and since refined sugar lacks vitamins your level of vitamin B will decrease relative to the amount of sugar you consume. This also endangers cell division, which is obviously not optimal. A classical example is shown by folic acid, which is necessary to break down alcohol in the body. Increased alcohol intake correlates directly to low levels of folic acid, and is one of the reasons why alcohol increases risk factors for breast cancer, an illness that can be drastically reduced by adequate folic acid supplementation.

A third account is that the breakdown of carbohydrates generates large quantities of free radicals, which are known to damage the DNA and can thus lead to cancer. Healthier alternatives to refined sugar such as raw cane sugar, agave syrup, maple syrup, honey, and date syrup contain high levels of antioxidants, which make them better options (39). An overall increase in calories in the diet is yet another possible culprit. As more energy is consumed, no matter the source, the bigger the risk is for developing malignancies. Refined sugar is highly calorific, and eating it can quickly lead to an excess intake of calories, especially if they're ingested via liquid form, as with soda.

THE MORE ENERGY CONSUMED, NO MATTER THE SOURCE, THE GREATER THE RISK OF DEVELOPING CANCER.

STUDIES THAT LINK SUGAR AND CANCER

● A Swedish study showed that the risk of developing uterine cancer increased by 40 percent in one fifth of individuals who consumed the most sugar, when compared to one fifth of individuals who consumed the least sugar (40).

● A very large study, comprised of 435,674 participants, showed the risk for throat cancer increased by 60 percent in one fifth of the individuals who consumed the most sugar compared to the fifth who consumed the least (41). According to the same study, the likelihood of rarer cancers, such as of the small intestine and mesothelioma, also increased when sugar was consumed.

● One tenth of those who eat the most sugar run an almost 40 percent higher risk of developing pancreatic cancer than the one tenth who eat the least of it (42). This is significant because it is one of the most serious types of cancer, with a high mortality rate and low survival expectancy. It's logical to conclude that the pancreas suffers when it deals with excess sugar, because it responds by producing and releasing insulin, the hormone most stimulated by sugar intake. The harder an organ must work, the more it becomes damaged. Several other studies concur with this observation (43, 44). Even refined fructose seems to increase the risk factor for pancreatic cancer (45).

● The risk for prostate cancer also increases with sugar consumption (46).

● Refined sugar increases the risk for breast cancer (47) and the same can be shown for cancer of the kidneys (48).

Some research shows that risk for colorectal cancer increases for someone who consumes large amounts of sugar, especially among men (49).

19

Forget Sports Drinks

THE WORDS "SPORTS DRINK" BRING BACK MEMORIES

Sports drinks remind me of my childhood during the 1970s, when a schoolmate's father introduced me to this type of beverage. The man was an elite tennis player, and he carried around pouches of powder that he mixed with water to drink during strenuous competitions. We boys would occasionally steal one of those pouches, but we never got the water-to-powder ratio quite right because the drink usually ended up tasting awful.

The next time sports drinks entered my consciousness was during my teenage years when I had begun working out intensely, and I started to use them quite liberally. The drinks didn't do much for my stamina, but they did put some weight on me. At seventeen, I was rather skinny, so this wasn't exactly a bad thing. Later on in my thirties, I was part owner of a badminton hall where we also sold sports drinks, and some of the regular players found them very useful during grueling tournaments, some of which could last a whole day. When the matches continued on into the next day, competitors found

it challenging to achieve their much-needed energy boost without these drinks.

Another set of customers at our hall happened to be middle-aged men, who rented time on the court by the hour. Even though their matches were shorter and less intense than those of upper-caliber and semi pro athletes, it wasn't unusual to see those weekend warriors down a can of sports drink right before the start of a game, making it more likely that the energy they expended on the court came from their drink, and not from the excess weight around their midriffs.

A SPORTS DRINK IS PURE SUGAR

Glucose and carbohydrate gels have the same effect on the body as sports drinks, in that they're an excellent way to replenish energy during a very strenuous workout. If you're an average exerciser, however, what you're using for energy is sugar instead of fat (50). Sports drinks are composed of water and simple sugars—mostly glucose—and some may add minerals acting as electrolytes to help delay muscle fatigue. Nevertheless, the mineral

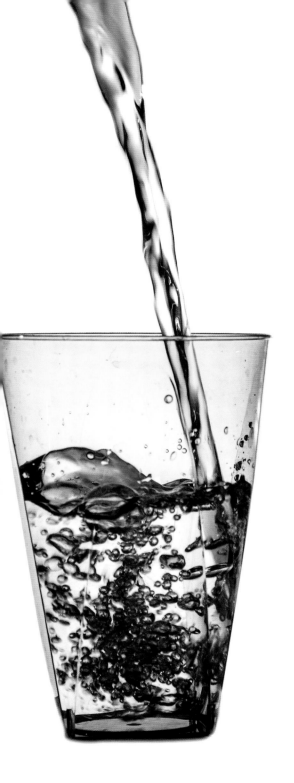

content is usually so low that a sports drink would be better labeled as a non carbonated soda. The GI value is high, and thus will push your blood sugar to levels that are neither healthy nor performance enhancing, that is, unless your workouts are atypically lengthy and/or grueling.

If you've eaten prior to your training session, then you already have an adequate supply of sugar in your bloodstream to keep energy at optimum levels throughout the exercise. Downing a sports drink will not improve your performance in any measurable way. In fact, it might release such large amounts of insulin that your blood sugar plummets rapidly and ends up lower than before your drank the sports drink, which would ultimately be detrimental to your performance.

DRINK WATER

If you do not regularly engage in strenuous physical activity, then water is your best bet. Be sure to drink cool, non carbonated water during your workout, as dehydration is bad for both your performance and your health. It can even be dangerous, as blood clots form more easily when you're dehydrated, and you increase your risk for heat stroke if you don't sweat enough during exertion. Cold water works well, as it brings the body's temperature down from the inside and helps empty the contents of the stomach, while restoring and keeping fluids in balance.

LET'S HEAR IT FOR TAP WATER!

Tap water is just as good as mineral water when you work out. Carbonation is not dangerous, but it decreases the rate at which you can drink, and you risk stomach upsets and excess gas in the intestines, which is unnecessary and uncomfortable. Last but not least, tap water, being free, is a far better deal than sports drinks.

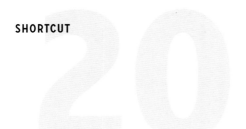

Making the Family Sugar-Free

SUGAR ADDICTED CHILDREN

I'm not preaching total sugar abstinence for everyone—it's only my own personal preference to want to avoid sugar as much as possible. As long as my children eat nutritious meals, I'm not worried about them having a bit of sugar here and there.

That being said, there are children who, sadly, have real problems with sugar and act out in the same destructive way I did as a child, when I took advantage of every opportunity to fill myself with sugar, and no cushion was left unturned at my house in my tireless pursuit of cookies, candy, and ice cream.

Today's society doesn't make it easy to cope with sugar-addicted children; there are occasions to indulge at every turn. It's not worth the effort to talk to children about their health or their weight, as there are very few things that can compete in their world with the lure of sugar. However, you might be able to bypass the problem by offering them really sweet fruit as an attractive replacement. Watermelon, persimmon, mango, oranges, mango, or granadilla (also called lemona) are all great substitutes for candy. Small bowls of pomegranate seeds or seedless grapes are both pleasing to the eye and tasty enough to make most kids happy. A few squares of dark chocolate also makes for a good treat, as it contains both fat and a satisfying sweet taste, and which—along with bitter and sour—acts as a natural appetite suppressant. Dried fruit is also a nourishing switch from candy, but do make a point of checking the fruit for any added sugar, and be mindful of serving sizes, as dried fruit, being a highly concentrated form of fruit, contains a lot more calories than fresh varieties.

BE THE FIRST ONE

If you'd like your family to eat less sugar, you must lead by example and remove sugar from your own diet and do your best to become as near to sugar-free as possible. It's common knowledge that children don't always do as their parents say, but they do imitate what they see. Don't think that if you carry candy in your purse that your children aren't going to want to eat some of it, so make sure to clean up your own act so you can be a role model to your kids.

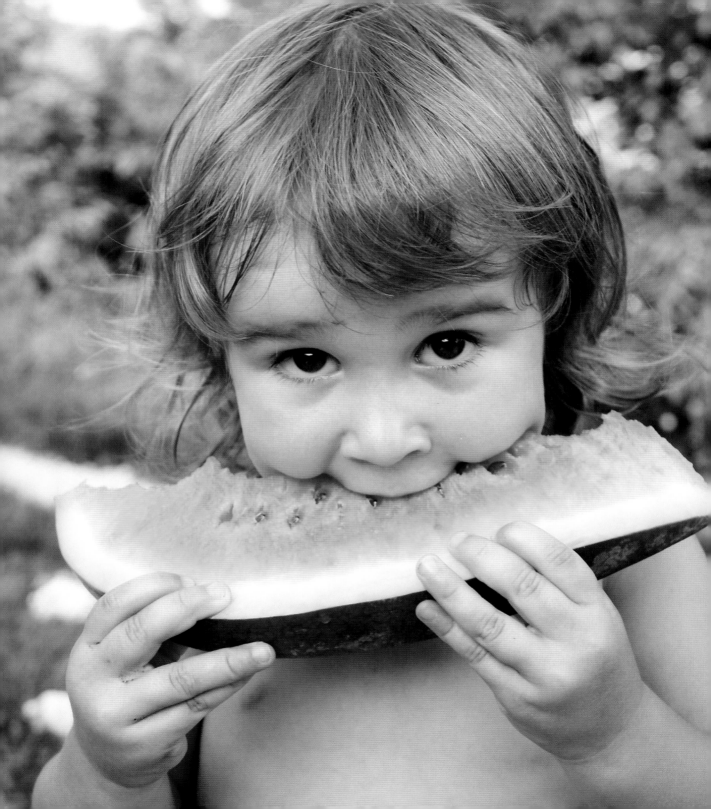

21

Less Stress and Less Sugar

HOW WE DIFFUSE STRESS

Stress can affect us in many ways, and most of us attempt to lessen it or deal with it by engaging in our favorite pastimes, such as listening to music, working out, practicing meditation, even eating food and drinking alcohol. Sugar also works for stress relief, albeit temporarily, since it releases endorphins in order to make the body produce serotonin, which has calming effects.

I have found that the very best way to relieve stress is through exercise. Make sure to get in at least half an hour of yoga, weight training, or running per day, and it will work wonders. Physical activity releases endorphins, and serotonin is made even while the muscles are at work, which helps keep you calm even when your life seems full of turmoil and obligations. Exercise is richly rewarding, by offering better physical fitness as well as psychological health.

MY OWN HISTORY OF STRESS

I'm often asked how I cope with having so many irons in the fire. I develop food products, write books, participate in fairs, own a nutritional center complete with a delicatessen, own a publishing company, give lectures, am a partner in a travel agency; I also try to have an active personal life that includes physical training, and spending time with family and friends. Sometimes when I look at my long list of commitments I also find myself wondering how everything comes together. The answer is that I have learned the importance of prioritizing, and I'll share my experience with you in hope that you might find it helpful.

My working life started early; I wanted to earn an income, but I also wanted to begin building capital to become the entrepreneur I always strived to be. I started out small by launching a variety of start-ups, but it wasn't until 2003, when I was invited to be on the panel of the Swedish television program, *Toppform* (*Top Fitness*), that things really took off.

In the beginning of my career I felt the need to accept every single opportunity that came my way. Suddenly I was receiving an avalanche of offers, and it was an awesome experience. Old habits die hard, however, and I kept accepting everything that was put in front of me. Not knowing how long this bounty would last I felt that I had to keep striking while the iron was hot.

Pretty soon my working life became a nightmare. I was a VP of a rapidly expanding publishing company and a much sought after lecturer. Things looked really grim when, in one single week of October 2003, my day planner showed that I had ten different speaking engagements booked across the country. I wanted to weep as I hit the road again after my seventh talk, when the plane I was riding to my next meeting flew over my home in Stockholm, without me being able to stop even for a short visit.

THE WRONG WAY TO HANDLE STRESS

This frantic pace of life continued for several more years until my stress started to manifest through physical symptoms such as heart palpitations and suppressed immune system. I noticed that I tended to feel confused; when I began experiencing muscle spasm in my arms, legs, and lips, I became convinced that I was suffering from a neurological disorder.

Multiple sclerosis, the dreadful disease that destroyed and ultimately took my mother's life, became an overwhelming and frightening concern to me when the feeling on the side of my right thigh disappeared, as well as in the tips of my fingers.

I somehow managed to fit a doctor's appointment into my crammed schedule, and thankfully the neurologist assured me that I did not show manifestations of the disease. He did suggest, however, that these symptoms might be psychosomatic signs of unrelieved stress. I had

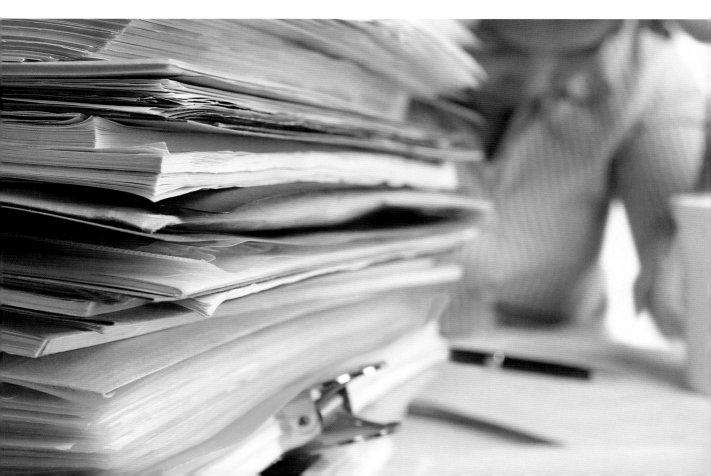

I HAVE CHANGED MY LIFESTYLE TO ONE THAT HAS ROOM FOR BOTH WORK AND PLAY.

always believed I could handle stress, but this was likely my body's way of telling me otherwise: it was sounding an alarm that I had finally reached the limit of what I was able to cope with.

I started by analyzing my dietary habits, and I quickly realized that I didn't eat as healthy as I should have, and, worst of all, I noticed that excess sugar had crept back into my life. My dependency on sugar hadn't returned with the urgency it once had when I was a kid trying to calm the anxiety brought on by my mother's illness, but I did eat sugar on a daily basis; I had established certain soothing yet unhealthy routines.

This became all too obvious at Christmastime, when my customers and clients offered me

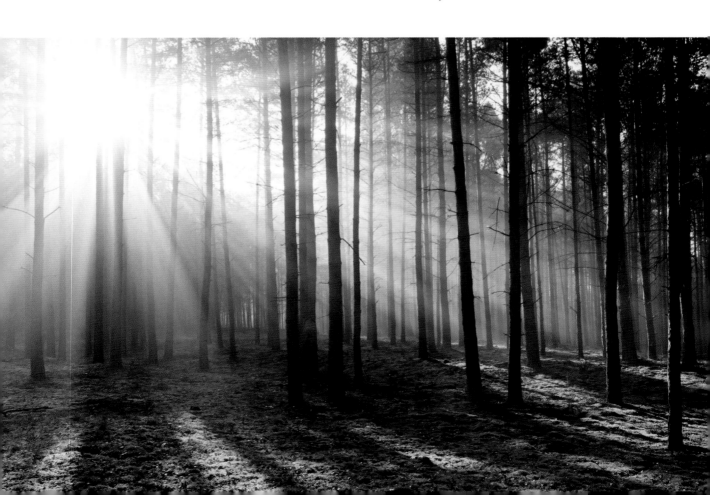

boxes of candy as holiday gifts, and I managed to clean the contents out of all of them.

I honestly can't recall how many candy boxes I was given, but my guess would be around 15 to 20 over a single holiday season. This uncontrolled sugar consumption, a reaction to my elevated stress level, made me put on twenty pounds: I went from weighing 75 kilograms (165 pounds) to 83.5 kilograms (185 pounds). My cheeks got rounder and my waistline strained against my belt when I finally realized this had to stop. It was time to enter a new phase and de-stress my life.

MY STRESS-FREE LIFE

To slim down and lower my risk factors for ill health (that my weight gain had brought on), the first step I took was to remove sugar from my life. Having read this far, you now know how sugar cravings come about, so the logical step was to stay sugar-free for a little over a week. I won't pretend it was easy; there were days I could have sold my soul for some sugar. To compensate for the void left by candy and to shift my focus away from sugar, I ramped up the intensity of my workouts. Once this strategy was in place, I needed to deal with what was at the root of this craving for sugar: my stress.

I started by taking a hard look at my schedule, and cut my engagements down to a more manageable three lectures per week. Many of my customers were disappointed, but it gave them the incentive to gather more participants to warrant my next visit. Instead of showing up in town three times a year, I now came once a year to three times my original audience. A DVD of my lectures was produced, and I agreed to let Swedish Television record and broadcast one of my lectures. In working this way, my message is communicated as effectively as before, the major difference being that I don't have to deal with frequent travel, late nights and all too early mornings, and long stretches of time spent away from home.

I also began arranging as many lectures as possible to be held during the week in order to free up my weekends. It's not by chance that the workweek has two free days at the end of it—we need this time to recuperate.

MY WONDERFUL PARTNERS

Early on I realized that a shared partnership is the right business model for me. It's better to own part of a business and concentrate on performing the tasks I'm good at, rather than to own it all and let some parts of the business slide. My fortes are in educating, inspiring, and informing people about good nutrition and healthy lifestyles; I fail miserably at administrative tasks. The answer was to join forces with a partner more suited to those types of responsibilities.

It usually takes less time and effort to accomplish something where you're inherently good at the task; you tend to be more effective and less stressed out by the job. In other words, don't tackle what you're ill equipped for! Get help for things you can't manage and if possible, delegate those tasks to lighten the load. Don't be afraid to ask for assistance and/or advice. People who are given responsibility usually step up and put their best foot forward, and it would have been impossible for me to be successfully involved in so many ventures had I not been able to depend on my partner's strengths, talents, and support.

The way I handle my lifestyle today gives me room for both work and play. It has taken me a few years to put it all into place, and I very nearly hit the wall, but I was lucky to learn from my mistakes and to have used them to redirect my life toward a more stress-free path. My present lifestyle makes it easier to abstain from sugar: I don't want sugar and don't feel any more cravings for sweets, so I'm able to stay at a healthy weight and enjoy life to its fullest.

SHORTCUT

22

Get a Good Night's Sleep and Have Less Sugar Cravings

SUGAR CONSUMPTION INCREASES WITH LACK OF SLEEP

Many people experience heightened cravings for sweets and get hungrier when they're sleep deprived. This is logical, since lack of sleep stimulates ghrelin production, thereby increasing appetite—especially for sweet tastes—and calorie consumption.

GHRELIN PRODUCTION IS STIMULATED BY LACK OF SLEEP. THIS INCREASES APPETITE AND CAN BRING ON HIGHER CALORIE INTAKE.

Even if you stay awake many hours over a 24-hour period and burn more calories in doing so, the overall end result will still be weight gain **(51)**. You need only to rise a few hours earlier in the morning and your increased appetite will lead you to consume more calories than your level of physical activity actually requires.

Another one of sleep deprivation's negative side effects is that it decreases the amount of leptin in the body, the hormone that keeps us satiated. Less leptin equates to a larger appetite.

It has also been shown that lack of sleep leads to less insulin sensitivity **(52)**, resulting in poor blood sugar balance. As you know, this is not good, because the risk for type 2 diabetes increases. All in all, a night of adequate sleep looks to be one of your best allies in controlling your blood sugar levels.

OTHER HORMONES ARE DISRUPTED

In addition to leptin levels falling, ghrelin levels increasing, and insulin production

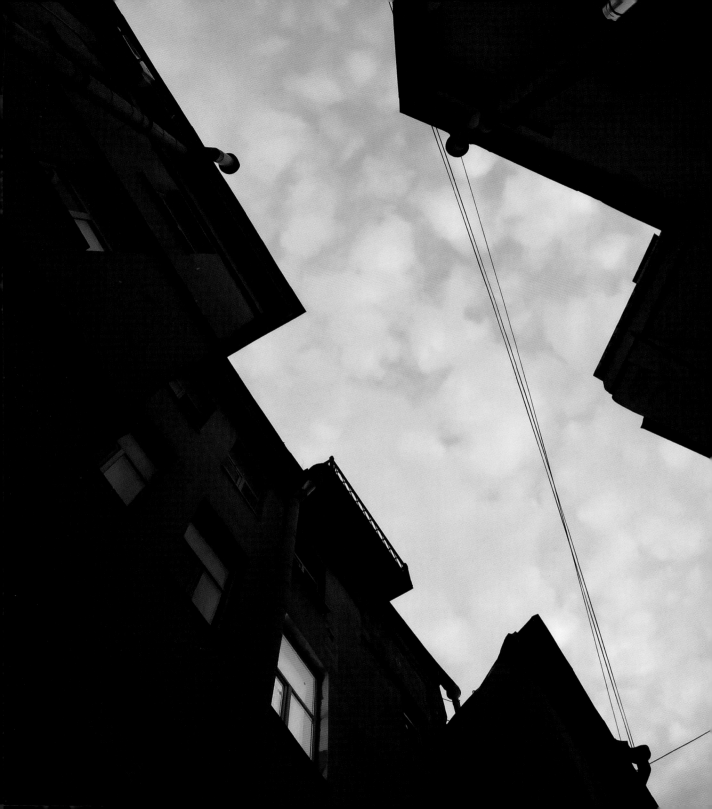

AVOID CAFFEINE RIGHT BEFORE BEDTIME.

adversely affected, cortisol levels go up during the night. Cortisol is a hormone that stimulates glucose formation in the liver, which increases blood sugar levels. It also stimulates the appetite as it increases the blood glucose level **(53)**. It's obvious then that higher levels of cortisol, along with sleep deprivation, are directly tied to higher risk of type 2 diabetes.

Research has shown that working the night shift, a systematic sleep disrupter,

increases ghrelin and reduces leptin, which, in tandem, rev up both appetite and cravings for sweets **(54)**.

JET LAGGED AND CRAVING SWEETS

A trip across several time zones now and then won't cause any adverse health issues, but things are different for the frequent flier. For airplane personnel, business travelers, and globe-trotting tourists, this type of travel poses a hazard to blood sugar balance. This happens whether the travel is one way out or a return flight over time zones **(55)**.

Since other causes of sleep deprivation have shown to be responsible for increased appetite and sugar cravings, the same probably holds true for jet lag, even if we don't yet have hard proof of it. Being familiar with how difficult it is for the body to balance its blood sugar during a spell of jet lag ought to be enough to be cautious around carbohydrates. It's not necessary to travel across time zones for a problem to surface, however, because any long trip can disturb sleep patterns, which is all it really takes to create a blood sugar problem **(56)**.

Apart from naps to help reestablish a healthy sleep schedule, exercise and a sound diet is the frequent flier's best friend.

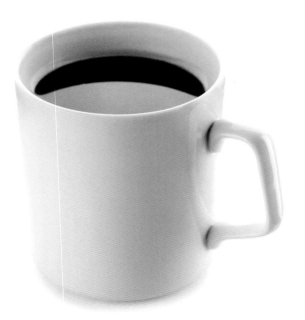

A SLEEP PRIMER

● Keep the bedroom as dark as possible, preferably with blackout drapes drawn over the windows. While it's easier to keep the room dark during the winter season, spring and summer can prove to be more problematic. Try draping a black T-shirt over your eyes if your room is still too light to achieve proper rest.

● Keep the bedroom cool. The right temperature varies according to each individual, but you should not perspire under the sheets. Throw different covers or quilts onto your bed depending on the season, and if weather permits, sleep with the window open to allow cool, fresh air to circulate.

● Make sure your environment is quiet at bedtime. Keep air-conditioning noise to a minimum, and make sure to turn off dripping taps and humming electronics.

● Avoid caffeine right before bedtime. We all know that there is caffeine in coffee, but don't forget that it's also found in most tea, colas, energy drinks, metabolic enhancers, and even hot cocoa.

● Organize your life around your biorhythm. There are many examples of night owls who, for some reason, need to start rising earlier than they'd like, and find themselves becoming more and more sleep deprived as weeks go by. The same problem occurs when early birds are forced to stay up past their naturally preferred bedtime. It's easier than you think to arrange work hours around your individual body clock, and it's to your advantage to choose your work or study habits to fit your sleep pattern, as your performance and overall well-being will benefit from it.

● Eat something light before going to bed. It can help you fall asleep faster, since fat and carbohydrates increase serotonin, which makes you drowsy.

● Don't bring your laptop to bed, and don't watch television in bed. Your brain will have difficulty relaxing if you keep it stimulated by electronic devices.

● If you don't get enough sleep during the workweek, make sure to compensate during the weekend when you can have a lie-in. Prioritize sleep to lessen the damage incurred by sleep deprivation.

Make sure your bed is cozy and comfortable. You'll spend a third of your life in bed, so it's worth every penny to buy the best bedding you can afford. Even the bed linen is important for good rest. There are many different materials available to you, and some people actually get better sleep if they machine press or iron their bed sheets.

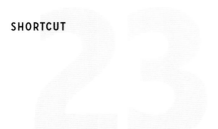

Exercise Yourself Free of Sugar

WORKOUTS INSTEAD OF WAFFLES

Humans are highly motivated to increase the brain's level of reward neurotransmitters. Dopamine is one of the most important neurotransmitters, as it promotes feelings of drive, purpose, and motivation. As mentioned earlier, it's released as soon as you eat sugar, and also when you're engaged in a pleasant activity.

This can be anything you enjoy, such as listening to music, going to the movies, having sex, or eating a good meal. Interest in shopping, gambling (both with computer games and casino games), alcohol, drugs (cocaine, for example), or the pleasure in the company of good friends all stem from the release of dopamine in the brain's reward center. Stimuli vary according to individual brain structure; some people prefer shopping to gaming, which means that a trip to the mall will release their dopamine.

Many activities that set off the release of dopamine are totally harmless, and some are even good for you; others are riskier. An interesting aspect of dopamine is that the body doesn't care how it's released, only that its level in the brain be kept high. That means that it becomes far easier to quell sugar cravings if you use other stimuli to release the dopamine, and exercise happens to be one of the more frequently tested stimuli.

WHAT KIND OF EXERCISE?

The guiding principle here is to participate in activities that you like. If you do something that's not enjoyable, then no dopamine will be released and your sugar cravings remain as strong as ever. Do you see the link?

You can also learn to enjoy certain activities when you begin to grasp how they work and how the brain-muscle connection is made. It most likely will not happen overnight, and it may take a few workouts. You'll also realize what type of exercise is unsuited to you, which you can then drop in order to pursue some other physical activity that you prefer.

Variation is often key to making exercise pleasurable, so don't get stuck on only one kind of activity. On page 114 you'll find more

THE GUIDING PRINCIPLE HERE
IS TO PARTICIPATE IN ACTIVITIES
YOU LIKE. IF YOU DON'T FIND
THEM ENJOYABLE, NO DOPAMINE
IS RELEASED AND YOUR SUGAR
CRAVINGS STAY THE SAME.

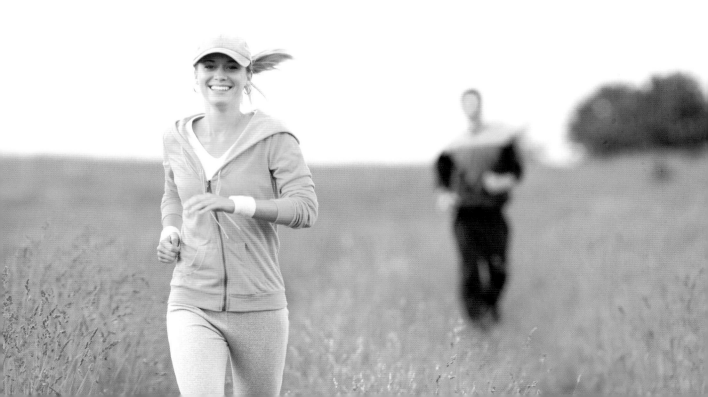

information about training and how often you should do it. You'll also read about how the act of exercising itself balances your blood sugar, which doubles the training's positive effect.

To break away from sugar addiction and bad eating habits without adding exercise to the mix is difficult. Once you're in the habit of being physically active, it becomes an integral part of your daily routine and will no longer feel like a chore but something you'll look forward to. When your cravings for sugar and fast food lessen, your eating habits improve. Eating better, in turn, enhances your physical performance and makes working out more fun. As you add more workouts your eating habits will continue to get better, and this positive loop spirals further onward and upward, giving you a new and revitalized life.

SEROTONIN STAYS LEVEL

By now you'll be aware that serotonin is the neurotransmitter that makes you feel happy and joyful, and that inversely, a lack of serotonin makes you unhappy and might even bring on depression. On page 50 you can find out about the blood sugar mechanism that raises the level of serotonin in the brain. In moderation it's a good thing, but when the effect is too intense, which could happen if you eat a bag of jellybeans, you'll only end up feeling sluggish and tired.

Exercise raises serotonin levels, contributing to a better quality of life and a happier outlook. This effect takes place by altering the balance between the amino acids leucine, isoleucine, valine, and tryptophan. The first three are also called grenade amino acids, and are among the few amino acids that can be used as fuel directly by the muscle fibers. Tryptophan, on the other hand, is the amino acid that the body uses to make serotonin.

When you put your muscles to work through exercise, some grenade amino acids in the blood are used up, which leads to there being more tryptophan in the blood than grenade amino acids. All four amino acids enter the brain by the same uptake mechanism, which means that there now will be a bigger uptake of tryptophan in the brain, and thus an increase in serotonin production.

This is one of the reasons why you feel calm and happy after exercising—the same feelings you seek when you eat sugar. Sugar produces identical changes in the blood as the aforementioned amino acids, and is why exercise is such an effective way to remove sugar cravings.

ENDORPHINS ARE RELEASED BY EXERCISE

The body has evolved a system for coping with pain. It's good to feel pain when something potentially harmful is happening to you; occasionally, however, the body perceives exertion through exercise as pain and something to avoid, so it creates a psychological block. Indeed, the first few minutes of taxing your muscles can hurt, but once you've warmed up and your body gets the message that you intend to continue with your activity, something happens: endorphins, which are powerful painkillers, are released and you can continue the workout without suffering too much discomfort.

The endorphins remain in your system for a while after the exercise session is over, giving you that calm and deep sleep you fall into after a satisfying workout. If you have been experiencing pain it is usually soothed, and if you've felt anxious, you will be calmer.

Eating sugar also stimulates endorphins, and that's why many people tend to self-medicate with candy, ice cream, and other sweets. Exercising quiets the need for endorphins, and this, together with dopamine and the serotonin, is the reason why exercise is your best friend if you want to cut out sugar from your life.

24

LCHQ for a Sugar-Free Life

LCHQ—MY LIFESTYLE

LCHQ is a lifestyle I have developed for everyone who, like me, aims to stay at a healthy, stable weight, to have plenty of stamina for exercise and work, and to fully enjoy his or her leisure time. Naturally, the food must also be delicious and healthy.

LCHQ is the acronym for Low-Carb, High-Quality, and is not a diet so much as a lifestyle tailored to anyone who values a better way of life. There is no calorie counting, yet the food is so satisfying that most overweight individuals will end up losing weight. The dishes are made from scratch with the best quality ingredients, and are completely sugar-free, so anybody dealing with a sweet tooth will benefit from following LCHQ.

The carbohydrate content is around 20 to 30 percent of the total calorie count, which is approximately half of what today's American typically consumes. This means LCHQ helps diminish blood sugar readings and insulin production, which is excellent for both health and weight control. The carbohydrate content is not as low as that recommended by LCHF followers (Low-Carb, High-Fat) who believe 5 to10 percent of daily calories is the optimal carbohydrate level. Such low amounts might foster low stamina and motivation for exercise, as well as general feelings of sadness or dejection, not to mention inferior nutrition. In my opinion, LCHQ is the ideal diet for most people. If you work out frequently, you'll need around 30 percent calories to come from carbohydrates, but if you're sedentary 20 percent is more in line with your requirements.

FAT AND LCHQ

With all due respect, carbohydrates are important, but the other nutrients play a critical role in our diet too. If you eat less of one type of nutrient, you'll have to make up for it by eating more of another. In our case, this means that 40 to 50 percent energy ought to be provided by fats, which is slightly above the 35 percent currently ingested by the average person.

Besides, our focus is on proven, healthy fats that aid in weight maintenance: omega-3s from fish, seafood and food crops like walnuts, rapeseed, and flax seed are all included.

Omega-3 fats appear to increase fat metabolism, all while providing excellent health benefits for the cardiovascular system and the brain.

Three servings of fatty fish per week, or something containing a little less fat such as white fish, mollusks (mussels, squid, or oysters), or seafood, have a daily place on the LCHQ menu.

Coconut oil and reasonable amounts of dairy fats are on the list of LCHQ foods too: short-and medium-chain fatty acids are now understood to be healthy for the heart and blood vessels; they appear to boost metabolism and to not be stored as fat.

Simply stated, these fats keep us slim, provided we consume them in reasonable amounts.

Nuts, seeds, olive and rapeseed oils, and avocados are other fatty foods belonging to the LCHQ lifestyle. They're made up of high amounts of mono-unsaturated fat, which is proven to protect against diabetes and certain forms of cancer, while being staples of the Mediterranean Diet,a regimen considered beneficial for cardiovascular health.

LCHQ recommends that you eat three servings of fatty fish a week.

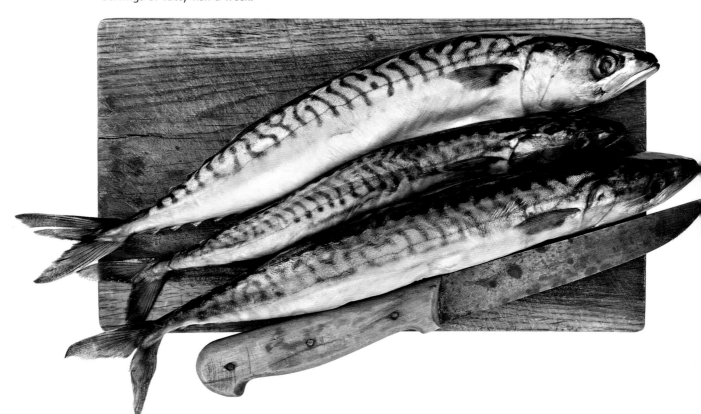

As fatty food goes, eggs are perfectly okay, but try to get Omega-3s that include the previously mentioned fatty acids, and less of the long-chain saturated fat—a fat to avoid. Long-chain fat is found in food like sausage, bacon, fatty meat, lard, hamburger, and similar products. When someone lauds bacon as healthy, please take it with a grain of salt. There's ample evidence that bacon is fattening, carcinogenic, and bad for cardiovascular health. Wild game is a far better alternative. It's not only a less fatty meat, but its fat is of a higher quality.

PROTEIN AND LCHQ

Protein is, per calorie, the most satiating nutrient, and also provides better recovery after you work out. It satisfies so well because it releases the stomach hormones CCK (cholecystokinin) and GLP-1 (glucagon-like peptid-1), which slows the rate of gastric emptying **(57)**.

A larger intake of protein decreases the hormone ghrelin, which leads to a lessened desire for sweets. Protein also seems to stimulate fat metabolism, and as it uses energy to convert fat, it raises the energy usage to complete this conversion.

A slower pace of emptying the stomach contents will level the blood glucose profile after a meal. Protein lowers the GI value on food it is eaten in tandem with, which sets off a lower insulin response. This is a very positive thing, in contrast to spiked insulin responses that promote fat storage, elevated blood lipids, high blood pressure, and increased risk factors for cancer and for type 2 diabetes.

Try to get your protein sources from meat such as wild game and low-fat cuts, or from fish, dairy products (cottage cheese, curd cheese, cheese, yogurt, and fermented milk), seafood, poultry, egg, legumes, and nuts. Likewise, you can find protein in root vegetables, vegetables, fruit, and berries, but know that the protein content of these foods is too low for us to subsist on alone. In LCHQ we recommend an intake of 20 to 40 percent protein.

EASY TO LIVE SUGAR-FREE

I seldom feel sugar cravings these days. Only after I've eaten refined sugar in one form or another—and this is something I do my best to avoid—will cravings rear their ugly head. Fruit, berries, honey, and other naturally sweetened foods, however, give me no trouble whatsoever.

It's easy to stay sugar-free with LCHQ. One reason is because your blood sugar stays in balance due to regular meals with low GI value and lower amounts of carbohydrates. Another reason is the relatively high intake of fats and protein to keep you energized and satiated, so you bypass those dips in energy that make the brain react by sending you strong urges to eat sugar and fat.

As you realize, LCHQ does not permit refined sugar, and it doesn't allow artificial sweeteners either. These tend to set off cravings for sweets in some people, and a good way to avoid these cravings is to stay clear of sweeteners altogether.

LCHQ encourages you to exercise regularly, and as you can see on page 82, physical activity is a sure way to lessen cravings.

A moderate amount of red wine is allowed when eating LCHQ, as it contains large amounts of antioxidants and other beneficial nutrients that release the dopamine you usually get from sugar.

LCHQ favors the use of spices, and we know that several of them (especially cinnamon) are good for balancing blood sugar, and thus contribute to easing sugar cravings and making a sugar-free lifestyle easy to follow.

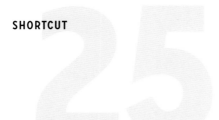

Reduce Sugar Cravings with Red Wine

REACH FOR A GLASS OF RED WINE INSTEAD OF CANDY

It might seem controversial to recommend drinking wine as a shortcut to a sugar-free life, especially when data from the *National Institutes of Health* found that 15 percent of the people living in the United States are considered "problem drinkers," and that of this 15 percent, 5 to 10 percent of males and 3 to 5 percent of females could be considered "alcoholics."* It should go without saying that this shortcut is not meant as an excuse to fall off the wagon for someone who might have trouble controlling his or her alcohol intake. Under these circumstances, there are far better shortcuts to explore.

However, if you're able to enjoy the occasional glass of red wine in moderation, this beverage has many proven health attributes, high among which is its notable blood sugar–lowering qualities that makes it a natural for inclusion in this book. Of all alcoholic drinks, red wine is the only one I recommend partaking in.

MODERATE DRINKERS OF RED WINE WEIGH LESS.

RED WINE AND ANTIOXIDANTS

Apart from alcohol, red wine contains many different antioxidants and active elements such as resveratrol, which is a powerful antioxidant shown to combat metabolic syndrome **(58)** (see page 103). In animal research, red wine has shown to prolong the life span of certain species, although it is not known if those results can be replicated in humans.

* Alcohol Addiction, "Alcohol Statistics," 2003–2012, http://www.alcoholaddiction.info/alcoholism-statistics.htm

THE DOPAMINE EFFECT

Research also shows that those who drink red wine in moderation tend to weigh less than non drinkers. Theories abound, one of the most common being that red wine drinkers generally follow a healthier lifestyle than others. But even when studies are controlled for this bias, red wine nevertheless exhibits beneficial weight-controlling characteristics.

During the body's metabolism of red wine, nearly half of 7 calories/gram are released as heat by the liver. In other words, wine contributes less fat-storing calories in the body than other foods, yet this still doesn't explain the wine's weight-loss effect. After all, in contrast to water, which is virtually calorie-free, red wine has calories, so logically it should increase fat storage.

Another hypothesis involves the aforementioned resveratrol, which seems to reduce fat storage at a cellular level. Yet again this comes up short as an explanation.

The current and prevailing theory is that red wine drinkers benefit from an added shot of dopamine in the brain, so are quicker to feel satiated after a meal. Thus, red wine seems to dull sugar cravings and make it easier to resist the lure of dessert or a bag of candy as a late evening snack. Without any conscious effort, red wine drinkers consume less sugar because they simply experience fewer cravings.

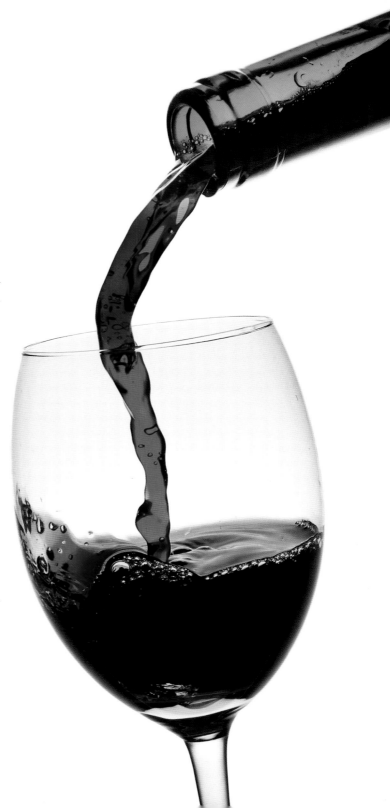

26

Allow Yourself Something Sweet Now and Then

CAN SUGAR EVER BE OKAY?

The fact is, sugar has effects that can be deemed positive, even beneficial. People who suffer from malnutrition, or hospital patients who have recently undergone surgical procedures and need to put on weight for their recovery, can be helped by the inclusion of sugar in their diet. However, it's imperative to combine this with foods replete with vitamins, antioxidants, fiber, and other elements that sugar lacks.

Many calorie-laden food-replacement products available for weight gain also have high sugar content. Part of the reason is to make these energy-dense products palatable while keeping their manufacture cheap; another reason is that it is a simple yet effective way to put on weight. These products are not meant to replace proper nourishment for any prolonged period, but are to be treated as a temporary calorie boost for a prescribed amount of time.

Another important aspect of eating sweets in moderation is that if somebody struggles to avoid sugar altogether, an inflexible attitude can easily backfire and lead back to intense sugar cravings. It's a constant battle to try to forego something entirely, so make the fight less fraught by allowing an indulgence from time to time.

SUGAR PROVIDES ALERTNESS, MOTIVATION, AND MEMORY

Each time I settle down to start writing a new manuscript, I always drink a glass of Coca-Cola—the original one, with sugar. Yes, you read that right! It has become a tradition by now. In my defense, the extent of my treat amounts to one can of soda per book, which indeed amounts to very

• •

RESEARCH SHOWS THAT SUGAR CONSUMPTION IMPROVES MEMORY.

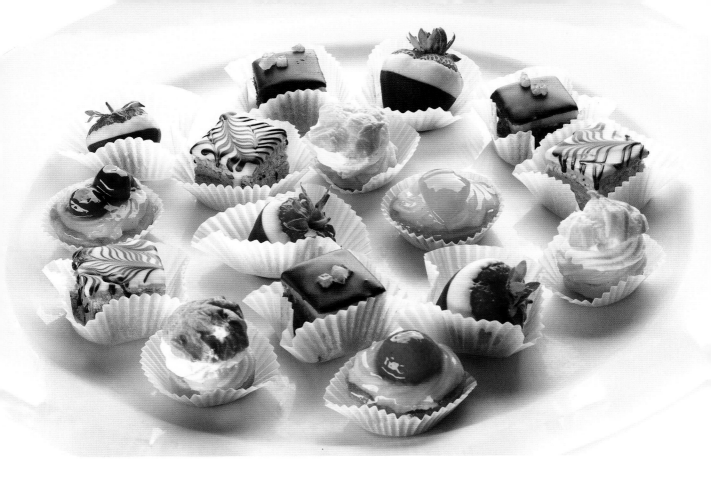

little sugar if you take the average amount of sugar in a can of soda over the days of one year—the usual amount of time it takes to complete a book.

I don't recall how this habit began, but it's obvious to me that sugar provides the energy and pep that helps me get started, since getting out of the starting blocks is often the most difficult part of any creative endeavor. Once the first chapter is written, that first hurdle cleared, the rest of the book flows easier. I'm sure caffeine enhances my motivation, as does the flood of dopamine released by the sugar in my drink.

If I were to down a quart instead of a regular glass of cola, my spiked serotonin level would make me tired and sluggish. However, the controlled manner in which I consume sugar—on very rare occasions and in limited quantities—has little to no detrimental effect on my health.

Likewise, research has shown that eating sugar improves memory. This biological function probably dates all the way back to the Stone Age, when it was beneficial for early man's survival and evolution to notice and remember exactly where those sweet tastes came from. It was crucial to locate and make use of this exhaustible source of energy and nourishment, which was the defining feature of sweet foods found in the wild.

27

Sugar by Any Other Name

IT'S ALL SUGAR

I understand that despite their best efforts, it's not easy for everyday consumers to recognize different ingredients on a label, to understand what they actually mean and how those ingredients impact the human body. Those ingredients often look and behave just like sugar, meaning that nutritionally, they're empty calories that do little else but raise blood sugar to unhealthy levels, and release loads of insulin.

Maltodextrin consists of long chains of glucose that aren't quite as long as those that make up starches; they're also more water-soluble, so they're often used in energy drinks or as a bulking agent in artificial sweeteners. Consequently, artificial sweeteners may contain large quantities of maltodextrin, which gives them an enormously elevated GI value and hardly makes them healthier than the sugar they're meant to replace. The only upside is that maltodextrin is very "fluffy" and weighs very little per teaspoon, which means that we don't ingest very much of it at a time.

Starches also add up to mostly empty calories. Many gluten-free products such as special breads and pastas are good examples of foods that are made up of little else than starch. Contrary to popular belief, it's about as healthy to eat these products as it is to eat a sugar-sprinkled cookie, so you should avoid all baked goods marketed as gluten-free.

• •

... INVERT SUGAR, FRUCTOSE, SACCHAROSE, SUCROSE, CORN SYRUP, DEXTRINS, MALTODEXTRIN, GLUCOSE SYRUP, FRUCTOSE SYRUP ...

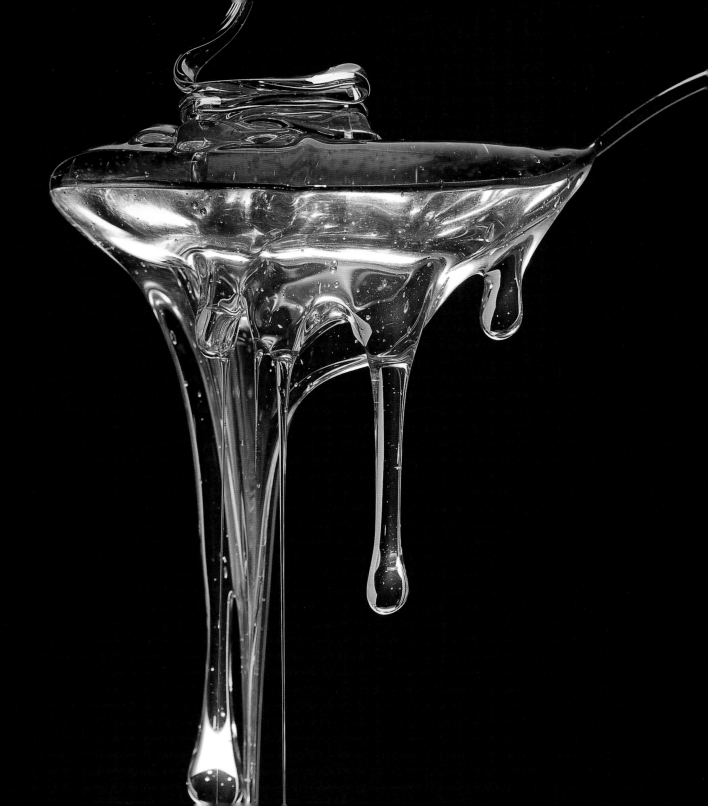

Corn syrup is another ingredient that turns up all over the place. The other day I actually saw it in beer.

Why would anyone add such an ingredient to a product that in its natural state only contains malt, hops, and water? To me, that's simply incomprehensible.

Maltos is an ingredient that reaches the highest GI value ever recorded for a sugar, which makes it far worse than sucrose for blood sugar balance, and as such it should be avoided.

READ THE INGREDIENT LABEL CAREFULLY

The ingredients in products are clearly listed on the nutrition label. This list includes all the ingredients contained within a product, and you should always go over this list if you're the least bit uncertain about what you've selected at the grocery store. Be aware that words such as "invert sugar," "fructose," "saccharose," "sucrose," "corn syrup," "dextrins," "maltodextrin," "glucose" "syrup," "grape sugar," "fructose," "starch," and "modified starch," are all simply sugar under different names.

On principle, none of them is any healthier than sucrose, and several of them are, in fact, worse.

Those sugar derivatives can be found in, but are not limited to: energy bars, protein powders, dehydrated sauces, pasta sauce, bread, drinks, snacks, convenience foods, and inferior protein sources such as reduced-price chicken breast. In some cases, the amount of sugar substitute is so small that it poses no risk to your health, but the fact that the food item had to be sweetened in order to make it palatable should warn you that you are eating an inferior product.

However, sometimes the amount of sweetener in a food is large enough to impact your health, which makes it all the more critical to show no leniency when dealing with these kinds of ingredients.

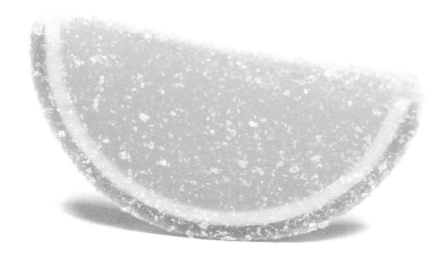

28

Better Blood Sugar Control with Water

WATER DILUTES THE RIGHT WAY

It's well known that drinking a glass of water with your meal will delay the emptying of the stomach, and promotes a better blood sugar response. The water content of food is similarly connected to your blood sugar, and also has an effect on sugar levels once the food has been ingested. So, the higher the food's water content, the lower the blood sugar, and vice versa.

It's easy to picture how this works. The lower the carbohydrate content in the gastric juices, the slower those carbohydrates are digested. They are for the most part absorbed together with the liquid in the small intestine, and the higher the liquid content, the longer the process. Besides, the liquid you drink dilutes the digestive enzymes in your mouth, stomach, and small intestine. These enzymes break down the starch from the food into glucose, and the longer this takes, the slower the uptake in the blood. There is nothing detrimental about this, as it doesn't decrease the nutritional uptake of the food; it only slows it down, which is good.

HORMONAL BALANCE

Your body releases a hormone called vasopressin when you're insufficiently hydrated. This hormone acts on the kidneys so that they conserve body fluid by concentrating the urine and decreasing the amount of urine that leaves the body. Vasopressin also elevates blood pressure by constricting arterioles, a logical step, since higher blood pressure is required to allow fluid to carry oxygen and nourishment to body cells, while simultaneously removing carbon dioxide and other waste products from the blood.

Consequently, the body produces more vasopressin when you only drink small amounts of water. New research has shown that this lowers insulin receptiveness and increases the risk for type 2 diabetes **(59)**. Thus, fluid intake is also critical to your hormone balance.

REPLACE INFERIOR CHOICES

There's obviously a positive effect on blood sugar when we opt to drink water with our

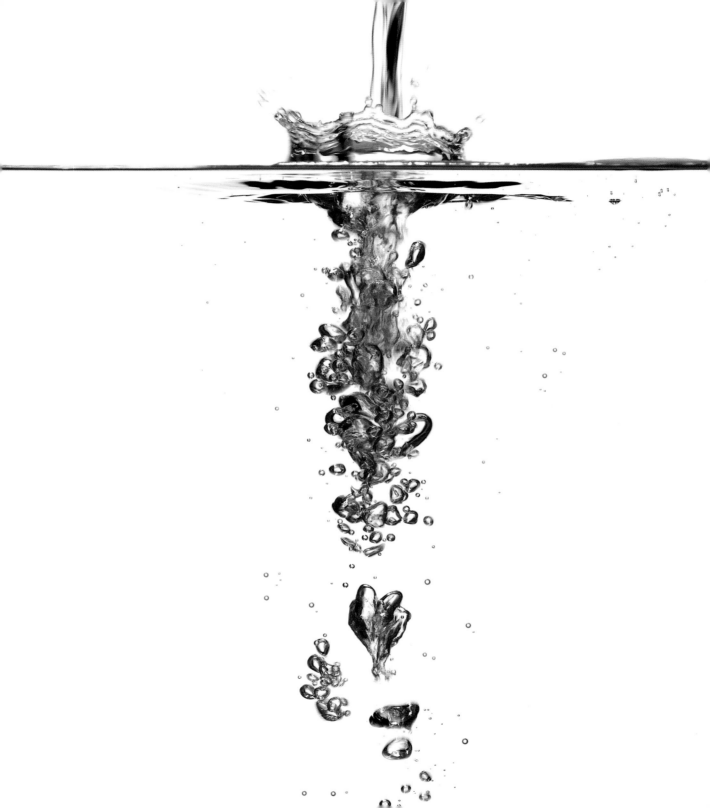

meal instead of juice, soda, beer, or other carbohydrate-rich beverages.

Drinking milk, light beer, and juice isn't detrimental to weight control and health, as long as we take them into account as part of the meal. To eat a full meal and then add on extra liquid carbohydrates will produce too much sugar in the blood, so it's hardly surprising that research has shown that when water takes the place of calorie-laden beverages, it lessens the risk of developing type 2 diabetes (60).

WATER INTAKE AND A HEALTHY LIFESTYLE GO TOGETHER

Research shows that people who drink a lot of water also lead healthier lifestyles and are less likely to become overweight (61). There are many reasons for this. We can, of course, presume that high water intake is synonymous with an active lifestyle, because we drink more water during and after a workout. However, we also know to a certain extent that water intake is linked to better health and more satiety—there are several studies showing a strong link between weight control and water intake.

HOW MUCH WATER IS ENOUGH?

The amount of water you should drink depends on the general makeup of your diet. Some people consume foods containing lots of natural fluid—fruit, vegetables, berries, roots, and yogurt can contain up to 90 percent water—in which case they don't need a lot of extra water.

If you're on a diet and are eating less food than you normally would, the need for fluids increases. Zero-calorie beverages like tea and coffee provide the necessary added liquid, and can be considered an adequate replacement for water. Naturally, the caffeine will stimulate the release of some of that fluid, but a good supply—70 to 90 percent—remains in the body.

Living in a warm climate and/or engaging in physical activity are also important factors to consider. Some people also have more active sweat glands and consequently lose more fluids.

In general, a liter (a quart) of pure drinking water is the minimum requirement for your body to function properly. You might need more according to circumstances—2 to 3 liters (half a gallon to three quarters of a gallon) if you jog on a warm summer's day, for instance—but for most of us, a daily intake of 1½ liter (51 fluid ounces) is plenty.

DRINK WATER AND LOSE WEIGHT

● In one study, 24 overweight participants were allowed to drink ½ liter (17 fluid ounces) of water thirty minutes before breakfast, or not drink anything at all. They were then allowed to eat without restriction at breakfast. The results indicated that those who drank water consumed 13 percent less calories than those who didn't drink anything (62).

● In another study, 14 participants (7 women, 7 men) drank ½ liter (17 fluid ounces) of water. When measured a short time later, their body energy expenditure had increased by 20 calories. Approximately 40 percent of that energy was used to raise the water's temperature from 22°C (71.6°F) to a body temperature of 37°C (98.6°F), so we might infer that cooler water from the refrigerator increases body energy expenditure to some extent (63).

● Another, larger study of 173 overweight women aged between 25 and 50, showed that a deliberate increase in water consumption to more than a liter (a quart) per day resulted in a weight loss of just over 2 kilograms (4 pounds) within a year (64).

RESEARCH SHOWS THAT PEOPLE WHO DRINK A LOT OF **WATER** LEAD HEALTHIER LIFESTYLES AND LESSEN THEIR RISK OF BECOMING OVERWEIGHT. THERE ARE MANY REASONS FOR THIS. WE CAN, OF COURSE, PRESUME THAT HIGH WATER INTAKE IS SYNONYMOUS WITH AN **ACTIVE LIFESTYLE**, BECAUSE WE DRINK MORE WATER DURING AND AFTER A WORKOUT.

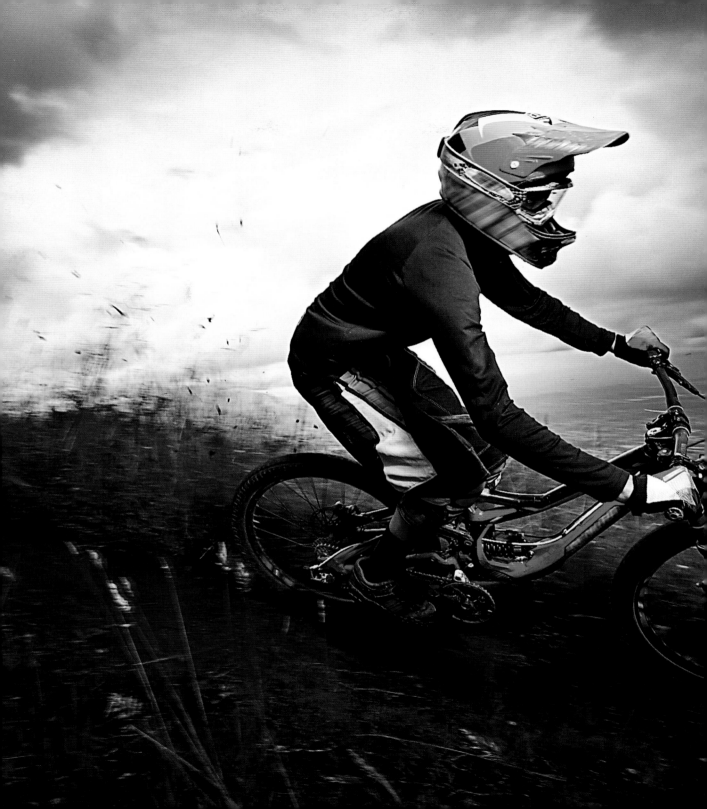

29

Avoid Prepared Foods and Mixes

A SHOCKING INSIGHT

Like many busy people today, I appreciate simple and convenient solutions, so I occasionally check out the ready-to-serve and premade food products for sale at the grocery store. Each time, however, I find myself baffled by the amount of sugar contained within these products. Why on earth is there sugar in ready-to-serve meatballs? Sauce for rice and pasta is other another type of product containing large amounts of sugar—sometimes so much of it that they turn out completely sticky.

It's better to buy ground meat and make meatballs from scratch, since they really don't take that much longer to cook, not to mention that they'll be far tastier and healthier for you. Keeping that in mind, I find it easy to forgo convenience foods and leave the path of least resistance. The time I spend making my own food will reward me many times over by making my life longer and healthier in the bargain.

IS IT THAT DIFFICULT?

Often, it's easier than you could ever imagine making your own food from scratch and without added sugar. To prepare a typical red sauce, for instance, you'll need to start with a can of crushed tomatoes. Mix its contents with some chicken or vegetable stock, a few cloves of crushed garlic, a tablespoon or so of tomato purée, a drizzle of olive oil, and a splash of red wine. Let this simmer gently for 10 minutes, and when time is up, add in some Italian herbs (oregano, basil, and the like) and some freshly ground black pepper to taste, and you will have a homemade, affordable, nutritious, sugar-free, not to mention absolutely delectable and vastly superior to any commercial brand tomato sauce for your pasta.

I believe that home cooking is more a question of attitude than anything else. I used to buy pancake mixes for my son until I googled a recipe for homemade pancakes—how difficult is that? I choose better ingredients too, by mixing whole meal flour that has quite a lot of rye flour in it, with organic eggs, non homogenized milk along with a dash of sea salt. You could not make better pancakes. Top them with some slightly thawed berries to make them even more delicious and boost their nutritional value.

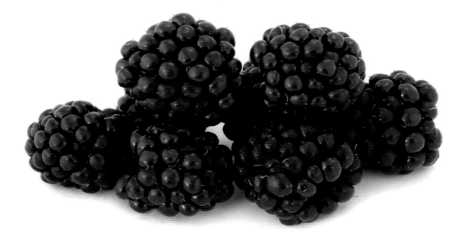

IF YOU HAVE A FREEZER

One main objection to cooking from scratch is that it's difficult to gauge how much food to prepare, and how to deal with the leftovers—food that might later spoil and need to be tossed out.

There's no need to throw anything away, since it's so easy, not to mention economical, to freeze extra servings. I am a big consumer of freezer bags. I fill them with single portions of food, then flatten them and stash them in the freezer, to reheat and eat at a later date (the contents of a flattened freezer bag defrost quicker than those frozen in a block).

All kinds of dishes, like roast chicken, tomato sauce, meatballs, hamburgers, and veggie burgers are great examples of foods suitable for freezing. They stay fresh in the refrigerator for quite a while, too. Sure, food can seem a bit dry and boring after three or four days' refrigeration, but it's certainly not unsafe to eat, provided that you cool and wrap the leftovers properly before refrigerating or freezing them.

Check out the food items below that I've black-listed. These are foods that usually contain a lot of added sugar if bought commercially, which I find are worth the effort to prepare from scratch. I'll admit that making homemade Swedish blood pudding is not a simple task, so maybe hamburgers are a more attractive option for you.

BLACKLISTED

Mayonnaise	Ketchup
Pancake & muffin/scone mixes	Peanut butter
Frozen meatballs	Freeze-dried banana
Swedish tube caviar	Candied fruit
Swedish blood pudding	Mustard
Pickled herring	Muesli
Cookies	Breads
Corn flakes/breakfast cereals	Yogurt
Pickled beets	
Whey butter	

101

30

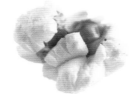

Snacks that Won't Upset the Blood Sugar Balance

ARE CHIPS A NO-NO?

For many people snacks are enjoyable, especially when Friday night rolls around and it's time to relax or socialize. A small weekly snack of a few chips is probably no big deal. Worse is when the snack is a food that can be mindlessly grazed on and a few pieces quickly turn into 200 grams (half a pound) of the stuff— that's when the negative health effects kick in.

Chips are deep-fried at very high temperatures, which generate the toxic substances acrolein and acrylamide **(65)**. Acrolein is also generated through smoking, and is strongly correlated to risk factors for a disease typically found in smokers: lung cancer **(66)**. Acrylamide, for its part, became infamous to Swedes when it was used as a sealant in the tunnel through an area called Hallandsåsen. It killed cows and poisoned workers, so it's hardly anything you want in your food. Acrylamide also produces malformed sperm in mice, which is another cause for concern **(67)**.

To get back to the topic of blood sugar: we know that all kinds of toxicity lower insulin sensitivity. All our regular body functions are diminished through smoking, drinking too much alcohol, eating too much; ingesting different toxic substances such as environmental toxins or even acrolein and acrylamide in chips. By that account we need to avoid them as much as possible.

There are many more reasons to avoid chips. Animal research has shown that they increase the risk for miscarriage. Rats who are fed chips produce less offspring **(68)**, and a larger amount of young are born malformed and underdeveloped. There has been no research yet to see if these findings can be applied to humans, but the very idea is frightening. What we do know is that eating 160 grams (5½ ounces) of chips per day over a period of four weeks increases the development of free radicals and inflammation in the body, so it would be harmful, even to humans **(69)**. The question is, just how harmful are they?

VEGETABLES AND DIP

Dip is not the first thing that comes to mind when we think of wholesome snacks, perhaps because it's typically served with chips.

To eat a dip with vegetables instead is another matter entirely. A dip based on the Swedish fermented cream *gräddfil*—which is similar to sour cream—does not elevate the blood sugar and it contains better-for-you fats, a total about-face from what was first believed.

For their part, vegetables are the world's most wholesome food, all categories included. They protect against many ailments such as weight gain, type 2 diabetes, cancer, cardiovascular disease, elevated blood pressure, cerebral vascular accidents, and stroke. Not to mention they're delicious, especially when eaten with a dip!

Simply cut broccoli, cauliflower, carrots, cucumber, endive leaves, sweet peppers, or celery into bite-size pieces and serve with the dip.

Although many ready-made spice mixtures pass muster, it's preferable of course to make your own dip from scratch.

CHEESE AND FRUIT

Cheese is a wholesome food. In the past it was believed that cheese was fattening and that it was responsible for cardiovascular problems. Cheese was also accused of causing lower insulin sensitivity and harming the blood sugar balance.

Today we know the opposite is true, that is, unless we overindulge. Cheese is very nourishing and is also a good source of selenium **(70)**, a nutrient often lacking in many people's diet.

Cheese is full of vitamin B12, vitamin D, protein, and good fats beneficial to brain health. Perhaps that's the reason why cheese has shown itself to aid cognitive function, the brain's outward measure of well-being **(71)**.

That insulin sensitivity is, if anything, improved by cheese consumption is interesting, and Norwegian research shows that cheese can even protect against metabolic syndrome in individuals who consume a lot of soda **(72)**. Metabolic syndrome is a collective term that refers to elevated blood pressure, elevated blood lipids, lowered HDL (the good cholesterol), and high fasting blood glucose. It's identical to high blood sugar, in that it increases the risk of developing type 2 diabetes.

Hard cheeses are better for you than the soft varieties, because it's protein that hardens the cheese, which also promotes satiety and balances the blood sugar.

So, why not cut up a few cheese sticks and serve them with fresh figs or a few slices of pear to make a perfectly nutritious and delicious snack?

POPCORN WORKS

Popcorn is a very wholesome and good-for-you snack. Popping it is easy, using organically grown corn kernels, coconut fat, and herb salt.

The kernels themselves are naturally whole grain, and contain large amounts of fiber and antioxidants such as lutein and zeaxanthin. The GI value is reasonably low and you'll get six times more popcorn than chips by volume, using a 100 gram (3½ ounces) serving size for comparison.

This makes popcorn far more satisfying than chips. Research has shown that a person will feel more satiated and satisfied after eating 100 grams (3½ ounces) of popcorn rather than just over 150 grams (5 ounces) of chips, which also happen to contain many more calories **(73)**. Try spicing up your popcorn with curry powder, black pepper, chili pepper, sea salt, or perhaps your own favorite seasoning.

It has been said that popcorn will collect in pouches (diverticula) in the colon and cause inflammation, but that belief has been debunked **(74)**.

Regardless, the very best snacks are nuts and seeds. They are in fact so wholesome that they deserve their very own chapter. Read about them in more detail on the next page!

31

Nuts and Seeds Balance Blood Sugar

NUTS AND SEEDS ARE SUPER FOODS

There are so many good things to say about nuts and seeds that it's difficult to know where to begin. It's easy to imagine, however, how our forefathers regularly enjoyed seeds and nuts in every conceivable way.

Nuts and seeds are among the most nutritious foods in existence. They're packed with protein, fats, fiber, vitamins, minerals, antioxidants, and other good-for-you nutrients.

Their energy content is very high, so as long as we eat them in moderate amounts they won't cause any weight gain. There are several reasons for this, one being that around 10 to 15 percent of energy goes straight through us and is not absorbed in the small intestine.

Another 10 percent or so is given off as heat by the liver when it's engaged in the task of processing food. Besides, nuts and seeds help us reach satiety quicker and in smaller quantities than other foods, so regular eaters of nuts and seeds tend to weigh less on average than other people **(75, 76)**.

The makeup of nuts and seeds also contributes to slower emptying of the stomach when you eat them with something else. Bread baked with nuts and seeds contain a lower GI value, and serving nuts alongside dried fruit produces a more drawn out blood sugar curve.

In this section I'll talk about a large variety of nuts and seeds that you can find in grocery stores, and I'll discuss their different characteristics and benefits.

ORAC is the acronym for Oxygen Radical Absorbance Capacity, a method used to measure the amount of antioxidants within 100 grams (3½ ounces) of produce. Nuts and seeds are very good sources of antioxidants, so I've chosen to include ORAC in their descriptions. A good supply of antioxidants is very important for proper insulin sensitivity and for healthy blood sugar balance.

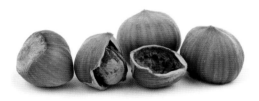

HAZELNUTS (FILBERTS)

Hazelnuts (also called filberts) contain a lot of minerals like magnesium, potassium, iron, calcium, and even selenium. Research shows that hazelnuts improve blood lipids **(77)** and protect against cardiovascular disease.

The antioxidants in hazelnuts decrease oxidized LDL (the bad cholesterol) **(78)**. This is a very important protective factor against cardiovascular disease, since oxidized LDL tends to stick to blood vessel walls.

Hazelnuts are also a good source of chromium. This mineral is vital in helping insulin keep blood sugar under control. You can read more about chromium on page 139, as it plays such an important part in controlling your blood sugar.

A study looking at the chromium content of Turkish hazelnuts showed that 1 kilogram (2 pounds) of hazelnuts contain all of 0.22–0.52 milligrams of chromium **(79)**. Therefore, 50 grams (2 ounces) of hazelnuts would provide you with 110–260 micrograms of chromium, which amply covers your daily requirement, as RDI (recommended daily intake) is a modest 40 micrograms. To eat a handful of hazelnuts per day is a smart move in looking after your blood sugar. Their ORAC is 9,500.

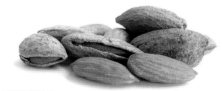

ALMONDS

The ORAC for almonds with the brown inner shell intact is a high 4,500. If almonds are blanched and the inner shell removed, then the antioxidant content is considerably lower.

The almonds are probably the most researched nut, studied for its effect

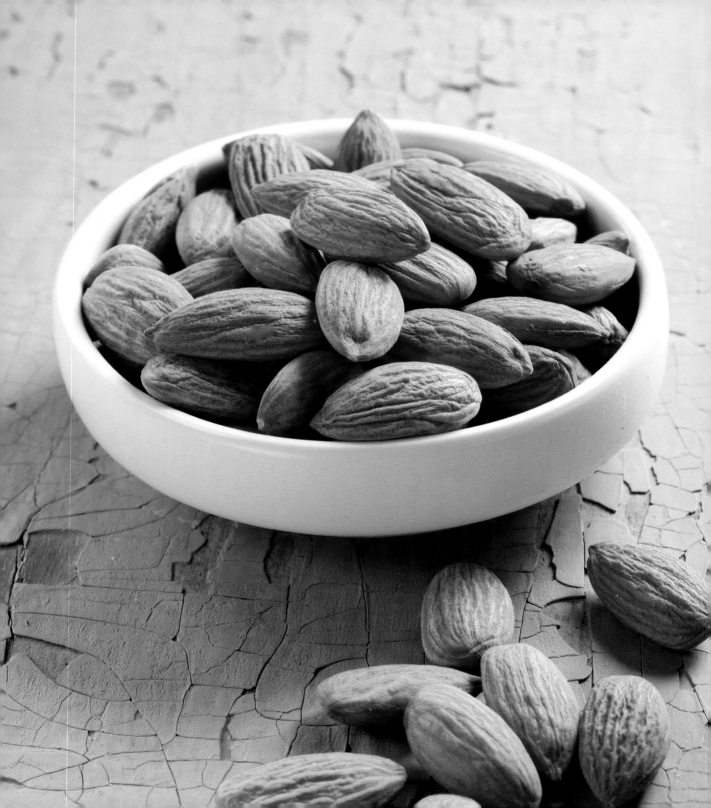

on blood sugar, because they're easy to procure, reasonably priced, and have shown themselves to be very effective.

A study of type 2 diabetics showed that as little as 28 grams (1 ounce) of almonds eaten together with a snack lowered the blood sugar response by 30 percent. In non diabetics it lowered the response by 7 percent (80). More almonds exert a larger effect on blood sugar, as demonstrated by a study showing a dose-dependent effect for 30 grams, 60 grams and 90 grams (1 ounce, 2.12 ounces, and 3.17 ounces) (81). Thus, the amount by which you want to reduce your blood sugar by is really a matter of how many almonds you're willing to eat, as 90 grams (3.17 ounces) of almonds are very filling and could be a meal in itself!

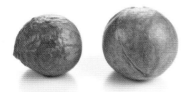

MACADAMIA NUTS

This is perhaps the most expensive and up market nut of them all. It's also delicious and good for cardiovascular health (82).

Macadamia nuts do lower the blood sugar response of food, but they are not the most nutritionally balanced. Their protein content is only 8 percent while fat content is a high 75 percent. They offer only traces of vitamins and minerals—the only nutrients worth mentioning being vitamin E and phosphorus: 100 grams (3½ ounces) of macadamia nuts contain 27 percent of the former and 34 percent of the latter. Antioxidant levels are quite low, so this nut should be treated as a delicacy, and not eaten solely for its nutritional value. Its ORAC is 1,700.

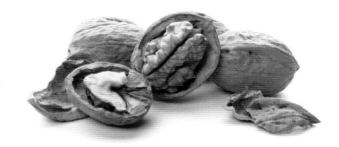

WALNUTS

These nuts' high content of omega-3 fatty acid ALA (alpha-linolenic acid) make them valuable to us all, but perhaps most especially to vegetarians.

New studies have also shown that walnuts improve human sperm quality. Eating just over 75 grams (2½ ounces) of walnuts per day over a period of 12 weeks improves sperm's vitality and motility, and it develops less abnormalities. There's no doubt that walnuts' good fats have a part to play in this, as do their high levels of antioxidants (83).

Another study showed that 15 grams (0.5 ounce) of walnuts, 7½ grams (0.26 ounce) of almonds and 7½ grams (0.26 ounce) of hazelnuts (filberts) taken together daily over 12 weeks lowered the blood's insulin level in individuals with metabolic syndrome (see page 103) (84). This is a sign that insulin sensitivity is positively impacted by the consumption of nuts, and will likewise be useful for keeping a person's blood sugar at a healthy level. Several more studies have replicated these findings, so diabetics who consume walnuts should show lower insulin levels (85).

Walnuts have also shown to improve the functioning of blood vessels (86), which decreases the risk of cardiovascular disease, and should also improve aerobic capacity in exercisers. Simply put, they will become fitter. Walnuts' ORAC is 13,500.

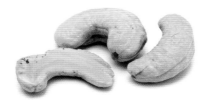

CASHEW NUTS

Cashews are one of the most common nuts available, and they're both tasty and relatively inexpensive. The carbohydrate content is somewhat elevated—around 30 percent—but the GI value is low, so it's still a good food; with a protein content of 18 percent and 43 percent fat, the cashew is a comparatively complete snack.

Cashews are also rich in iron and zinc, and a 100 gram (3½ ounce) serving provides approximately half the daily requirement of both minerals.

Other minerals provided by cashews are selenium and magnesium. Surprisingly, roasting cashews has shown to increase their antioxidant level (87). Cashews are good additions to stir-fries, but you shouldn't hesitate to sprinkle them on any of your other meals, as they provide extra nutrition and lower the GI value of the entire dish. The ORAC for raw cashew nuts is 1,950.

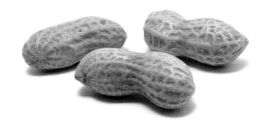

PEANUTS

The ORAC for peanuts is a respectable 3,100, and like other nuts they slow down gastric emptying (88). However, they are comparatively inferior from a nutritional standpoint.

Botanically speaking the peanut is a legume, and in order to be edible and digestible it needs to be roasted first. Roasted peanuts contain high levels of AGE (advanced glycated end products) and ALE (advanced lipoxidation end products), which are the damaged carbohydrates and fats linked to lowered insulin sensitivity, and could lead to higher blood sugar levels, and in some cases, type 2 diabetes (89). Because of this, it's prudent to limit one's consumption of roasted peanuts, such as in peanut butter.

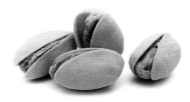

PISTACHIO NUTS

Pistachios' ORAC is around 7,500, which is a good value and places the pistachio nut at the top. Its green color indicates high antioxidant content, but doesn't reveal much of its other qualities.

However, research has shown that as little as 42 grams (1½ ounces) of pistachio nuts significantly hold back blood sugar increases in a diabetic person for up to two hours after a meal (90). Not surprisingly, 70 grams (2½ ounces), is even more impactful. Further, the same study showed that the addition of nuts did not result in weight gain for the study participants. Another study showed that pistachio nuts lowered the GI value of other foods eaten together with the nuts (91). This held true for all three amounts of nuts eaten—28 grams, 56 grams, and 84 grams (1 ounce, 2 ounces, and 3 ounces)—which means that it's not necessary to eat large amounts of pistachios to reach a blood sugar balancing effect.

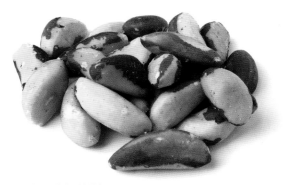

BRAZIL NUTS

The ORAC of Brazil nuts is a modest 1,400, but this is balanced by the selenium content that boosts your own antioxidant production—a property that isn't discernible in the ORAC measure.

Brazil nuts have an abundance of squalene, a fat that is also found in great amounts in shark liver oil (a source that naturally must be avoided due to ecological concerns). Research indicates that squalene can protect against cancer while acting as an antioxidant **(92)**, another aspect that doesn't show up in the ORAC measure. The truth is that Brazil nuts are the best source of squalene compared to other nuts **(93)**.

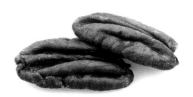

PECAN NUTS

The ORAC for pecan nuts is 18,000, which makes them the most antioxidant-rich nuts around. Fat content is high, making them very effective in slowing down blood sugar uptake after a meal. Try pairing pecans with bananas in a snack; they complement each other well and make you feel full for a long time.

Pecan nuts are known to lower the level of LDL in the blood. LDL can, as mentioned earlier, attach itself to blood vessel walls if oxidized, something pecan nuts offer protection against. These nuts can be considered a two-pronged guard against cardiovascular disease.

As if that weren't enough, it looks as though pecans might offer protection to the nervous system as we age and grow older, which helps preserve muscle strength—a necessity for moving about effectively and injury-free, and keeping our blood sugar under control.

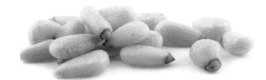

PINE NUTS

While their ORAC reads a low 720, pine nuts are a very good alternative for those who cannot eat nuts. Botanically, the pine nut is a seed and is therefore usually well tolerated by everyone, including those who suffer from allergies to nuts.

Fat, protein, and carbohydrate content is similar to any other nut, with one exception: 25 grams (1 ounce) of pine nuts provides the daily requirement of manganese. (This underlines the point that a mix of different nuts and seeds is the best the way to derive nutritional benefits from our diet.) They are perfect roasted, sprinkled over salads for a delicious taste, and to achieve blood sugar balance.

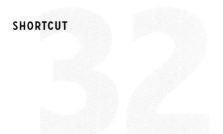

Fat and Blood Sugar

FAT IS OUR FRIEND

From a general standpoint, we can confidently say that fat is good for keeping blood sugar in check. Fat releases CCK (cholesystokinin), the digestive hormone that slows the emptying of the stomach, and therefore brings down the rate at which carbohydrates reach the small intestine.

While all fats have this positive effect on digestion, some of them are better than others with respect to overall nutritional quality and insulin sensitivity. Thanks to our increased understanding about this substance, we recommend that each meal contains some fat. Popular diets of the '80s and '90s that emphasized low-fat or fat-free foods brought about constant blood sugar swings; people who followed those regimens found it difficult to feel satisfied, and many were besieged by sugar cravings and an ever increasing appetite.

Here is a primer on fats, and how they impact blood sugar.

MONOUNSATURATED FAT

When glucose enters the bloodstream and becomes blood sugar, the body always reacts by releasing insulin. The insulin swims in the blood and binds to the body's insulin receptors. These receptors are located on the outside of liver cells, muscle tissue cells, fat cells, kidney cells, and brain cells—to mention only a few places—where they function as keyholes; the insulin is the key.

When the insulin binds to a receptor, it unlocks the cell to which it belongs, and a signal passes from the cell's receptor to the cell membrane. Because the cell membrane is mostly comprised of fat, the type of fat you consume has a major impact here.

For example, if you eat a lot of monounsaturated fat, your cell membranes become soft, which helps them retain their correct shape and stay healthy. The insulin receptor signal passes easily into the cell, telling it that it's time to take up glucose. This is what we call insulin sensitivity, and for this reason monounsaturated fat is good for blood sugar balance.

IMPROVING THE BRAIN'S INSULIN SENSITIVITY

It has only recently come to light how critical it is to have optimum insulin sensitivity, even in the brain. If this sensitivity is lowered, an individual will tend to gain weight, and it may become increasingly difficult for this person to control his or her appetite. Further, brain functions begin to suffer—cognitive processes are damaged and memory becomes impaired **(94)**.

There are many indications that dementia-like ailments, such as Alzheimer's disease, are caused in part by impaired insulin sensitivity in the brain. As insulin behaves the same way in the brain as in all other body tissues, it's not far-fetched to infer that brain sensitivity is directly tied to the fats we choose to eat. Monounsaturated fat seems to be the best option for keeping mental faculties sharp **(95)**.

LONG-CHAIN SATURATED FAT

You can eat moderate amounts of long-chain saturated fat, found primarily in sausages, bacon, hamburgers, lard, and other fatty animal products. If you eat too much of them, however, your insulin sensitivity will decrease **(96)**. If you omit mono-unsaturated fats and the omega-3 fats from your diet in favor of long-chain saturated fat, your cell membranes will in time become rigid and brittle.

This is perfectly logical: your cells are surrounded by membranes that are built from the fats you consume; if you eat hard long-chain fats, your cell membranes become hard. As I'm sure you're aware of by now after reading the paragraph about monounsaturated fats, this is a problem.

Hard cell membranes allow insulin to bind to its receptors, but the signal from the receptor has trouble penetrating into the cell. Consequently, blood sugar doesn't decrease as it should, which in the long run could lead to serious health problems like type 2 diabetes.

This can affect insulin sensitivity in even a short amount of time, so you need to keep an eye on how much saturated fat from animal products you eat. Lean meat and wild game are preferable choices to fatty, processed, or marbled meat. Short-and medium-chain fats—plentiful in dairy products and coconut—do not pose the same health risks, as these function as a fuel for cell membranes, rather than as building blocks.

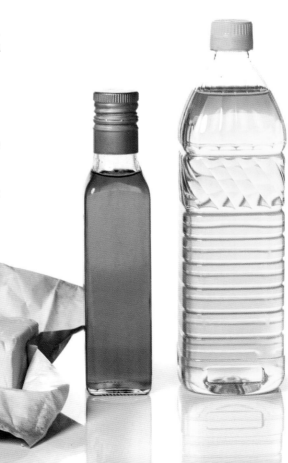

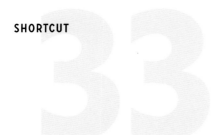

Protein and Blood Sugar

THE WHOLESOME BRAKE SHOE

Like fat, protein is a nutritious substance that slows the emptying of the stomach and balances blood sugar. It sets off the release of the digestive hormone cholesystokinin (CCK).

Because of this, adding protein to a meal brings about a slower blood sugar curve and longer satiety **(97)**. It can also increase one's power of concentration and improve memory **(98)**. Therefore, no meal is complete without protein. No matter your age or sex, what profession or studies or other pursuits you're engaged in, a certain amount of protein in every meal will give you a better quality of life with improved cognitive function and a happier disposition. As you've read in the Shortcut about LCHQ on page 87, between 20 to 40 percent of protein is enough. That means that in order for you to feel your best, between 20 and 40 percent of your total calories should come from protein.

PROTEIN QUALITY PLAYS A ROLE

Different proteins contain different types of amino acids. There are approximately 20 amino acids in proteins, and as they all serve different functions in the body, it's fully conceivable that they may each exert influence on insulin sensitivity and blood sugar in different ways.

Proteins break down into peptides (small amino acid stumps), which are taken up relatively intact. These peptides are usually unique to the food from which they are derived and have interesting physiological properties.

Fish protein in particular is a nutrient that seems to have a very beneficial influence on insulin sensitivity. In one study, 34 participants ate 3 grams (0.11 ounce) of fish protein per day over a period of four weeks; their amount of fish protein was then upped to 6 grams (0.21 ounce) per day during the next four weeks, the equivalent to 15 to 30 grams (½ to 1 ounce) of fish daily.

Several effects were noticed. Fasting glucose levels decreased and blood sugar levels dropped within two hours of finishing the meal. Insulin and LDL (the bad cholesterol) levels dropped also **(99)**.

It should be noted that even with a low dose and only after four weeks, that muscle mass had increased and adipose tissue had decreased in the study's participants.

EAT RATHER THAN DRINK YOUR PROTEIN

Today, many people consume protein drinks in the hopes of boosting their quality of nutrition in general, and achieving higher protein intake specifically. There is nothing really wrong with this, but research shows that protein obtained in the form of whole foods satiates more and improves blood sugar response because it slows down the emptying of the stomach.

In one study, 15 teenagers were given a breakfast of either 48 grams of liquid protein or the same amount in whole foods. After four hours, the participants who drank their protein were a lot hungrier than the participants who ate theirs whole **(100)**. This isn't surprising, since the liquid protein passed into the stomach at a quicker rate, and you only have to do a small calculation to realize just how much food you need to eat in order to get 48 grams of protein—it corresponds to almost 250 grams (9 ounces) of chicken breast, compared to 6 to 7 deciliters (23 fluid ounces) of a protein drink.

Protein powder can be appropriate after a workout, because the protein can easily be digested soon after physical activity for quick recovery and added muscle mass.

I prefer whole foods to protein powder when it comes to daily meals, because there is so much more nutrition in whole foods and it is fresher and healthier. Protein powder also has the capacity to produce AGE (Advanced Glycated End Products) and ALE (Advanced Lipid Glycation) and have, in fact, the highest content of these damaged nutrients among any food **(101)**.

AGEs and ALEs can best be described as old nutrients that have passed their prime and are becoming waste products that cause inflammation in the body. For safety's sake, my recommendation is to consume no more than a few portions of protein powder weekly.

FISH PROTEIN HAS GOOD EFFECTS ON INSULIN SENSITIVITY.

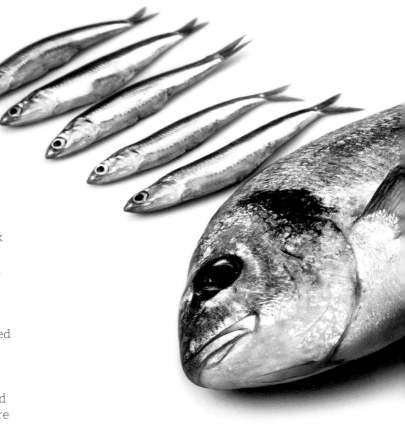

34

Exercise for Stable Blood Sugar

FAT BURNS SLOWLY ALL ON ITS OWN

Did you know that every step you take and every move you make balances your blood sugar? The mechanics are simple: A working muscle needs energy to function, which is provided from the surrounding blood. Exercise increases the release of free fatty acids from the fat cells.

Fat cells release fatty acids instead of storing them, and the longer you exercise, the more free fatty acids are released into the blood and reach the muscle mass. The more free fatty acids are in the blood, the more of them your muscles are able to take up and utilize for energy. This process has its limits, however, and the body can only burn fat up to a point. Since your working muscles still need more energy than fatty acids can provide, that's when carbohydrates enter the picture.

CARBOHYDRATES NEED SOME ASSISTANCE

A very ingenious process takes place in order for muscles to access glucose from the blood: as soon as a muscle is put to work during an activity, it starts to generate a protein called GLUT-4 (glucose transport protein 4). In simple terms, it's a protein that enables glucose to pass through the muscle cell membrane so that it may be used as energy.

This means exercise has a direct blood sugar reducing role, and it's why you can work off some excess weight if you've overindulged on unhealthy foods. It's the same protein that is made when insulin binds to its receptor and imparts its blood sugar–lowering effect.

• •

EXERCISE SUCH AS JOGGING, BIKING, AND SWIMMING IS EXCELLENT TO ENSURE GOOD INSULIN SENSITIVITY.

On a practical level, exercise and insulin are wholly interchangeable, as the more you exercise, the less insulin you need to keep your blood sugar in check. That's also why you need to eat several small meals on days when you exercise compared to the days when you don't.

Another helper in muscles' uptake of glucose is nitric oxide, which increases blood flow in the body, which in turn lowers blood pressure and facilitates the transport of glucose to the muscles. The same beneficial effect can be had through exercise **(102)**.

MORE ADVANTAGES TO EXERCISE

Apart from softening spikes in blood sugar, exercise automatically lowers insulin levels. This has good implications for fitness, weight, and health, as insulin can be problematic in many cases.

First, insulin increases fat storage, so less amounts of insulin facilitate weight loss and also make it easier to avoid regaining lost weight. It goes without saying that it's not a fluke that exercise is considered one of the most important strategies for controlling body weight.

Second, insulin stimulates the conversion of carbohydrates into fat, which produces increased blood lipids and adipose tissue—otherwise known as body fat.

Third, the insulin regulating mechanism in your cells simply becomes exhausted if it always has too much to handle. In the long run, it will lead toward lowered insulin sensitivity, and possibly even type 2 diabetes, so it's critical for those who want to get rid of diabetes to lower their insulin level. In so doing, insulin sensitivity normalizes and exercise is one of the best methods by which to achieve this.

Fourth, insulin stimulates cell division, which increases the risk of cancer and premature aging. It appears that the cells have a certain pre programmed amount of cell division for the duration of their life span, after which they stop and die. The higher your insulin in your blood, the faster this cell division takes place, and the quicker you age. One mechanism that prolongs cells' life span seems to be, again, exercise.

WHAT TYPE OF EXERCISE IS BEST?

I know people who have been diagnosed with type 1 diabetes—the kind of diabetes where there is no insulin production whatsoever—who do not need to take insulin injections because they exercise so vigorously.

I don't necessarily believe that amount of exercise is healthy over the long haul, because such high levels of activity also leave the body vulnerable to excessive wear and tear.

EXERCISE IS GOOD FOR INSULIN SENSITIVITY

Research shows that high intensive interval training is very good for insulin sensitivity **(103)**.

Martial arts, Spinning, and soccer are examples of exercise containing elements of high-intensity interval training.

The more cardio-oriented forms of exercise such as running, biking, and swimming all benefit insulin sensitivity, and will also increase mitochondrial density **(104)**. Metabolic syndrome is characterized by a decrease in the amount of mitochondria in the muscles, so exercise is an effective way of reversing this trend.

Later research shows that weight training is also excellent for increasing insulin sensitivity **(105)**.

However, it clearly illustrates how effective physical activity can be. Naturally, you're free to choose your exercise regimen according to your tastes and preferences, as my point is that you should do what you enjoy. The most important thing here is to do something.

As a rule of thumb, I suggest performing three training sessions, lasting 45 minutes each, every week; this is an absolute minimum to notice measurable effects on insulin sensitivity. Less exercise is not a waste of course, but my recommended workout is only a little extra effort for such a handsome payoff!

If you can spare the time, aim for one hour of exercise per day; I believe this to be ideal for optimum blood sugar balance. You can also work out a little less strenuously, since you have upped the frequency of your physical activity. Very strenuous training has, in practice, shown to lower insulin sensitivity momentarily, because muscles sustain more damage from the effort of intense exercise.

It seems that the very best training is a mix of different types of exercise. You will benefit from both aerobic activity (when the muscles use oxygen) and its anaerobic counterpart (when they work without oxygen); that is, you should engage in some power walking, for instance, along with some weight training. Adding variety to your activities lessens the likelihood of burnout and injury, and also makes exercising more fun.

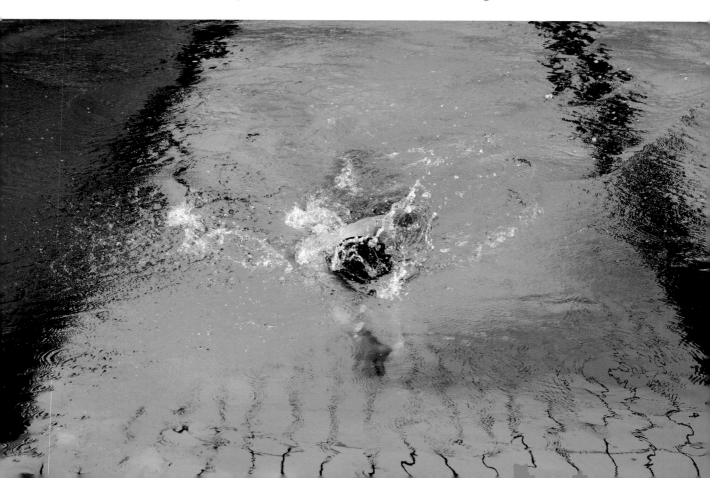

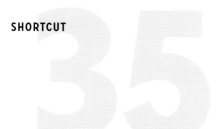

Legumes—Blood Balance's Royalty

UNIQUE COMBINATION

Lentils, peas, and beans all belong to the legume family, as do peanuts. What makes legumes unique is their high content of both carbohydrate and protein. This is a highly unusual combination among foods; the only other edibles that come close are seeds and nuts, although legumes have an even better balanced nutritional content.

By adding a little oil or some other healthy source of fat, such as avocado, you can prepare a nutritionally complete dish from legumes.

High protein content is one of the reasons why legumes are so good for our blood sugar. It slows gastric emptying, and together with its compact structure and high fiber content, I declare legumes to be the royalty of the balanced blood sugar world.

Legumes have low GI value when eaten alone; when eaten as part of a complete meal they lower the GI value of the entire dish. Add legumes to a salad, or let them enrich a stew and they will help balance out your blood sugar level. Even mashed legumes, in the form of hummus, or a pot of long-simmered beans or lentils, have low GI value, which is surprising since the structure of the legume itself has been destroyed. The secret lies in their anti-nutrients.

ANTI-NUTRIENTS LOWER GI VALUE

Legumes have a natural defense mechanism protecting them from being eaten. Biologically, they act like a seed. If they're consumed, they never have a chance to end up intact in the soil, thus making them unable to take root. In the form of seed, however, they're full of nutrition, and a lot of energy and nutritive elements are necessary to produce roots and gradually grow into a new plant.

So in order to protect themselves against being consumed, they have evolved to produce something called anti-nutrients, which are a fascinating group of compounds that interfere with the enzymes that break down nutrients.

The result is that, if you eat a meal that contains legumes, it will take a longer time to digest it. Some of the food is not absorbed,

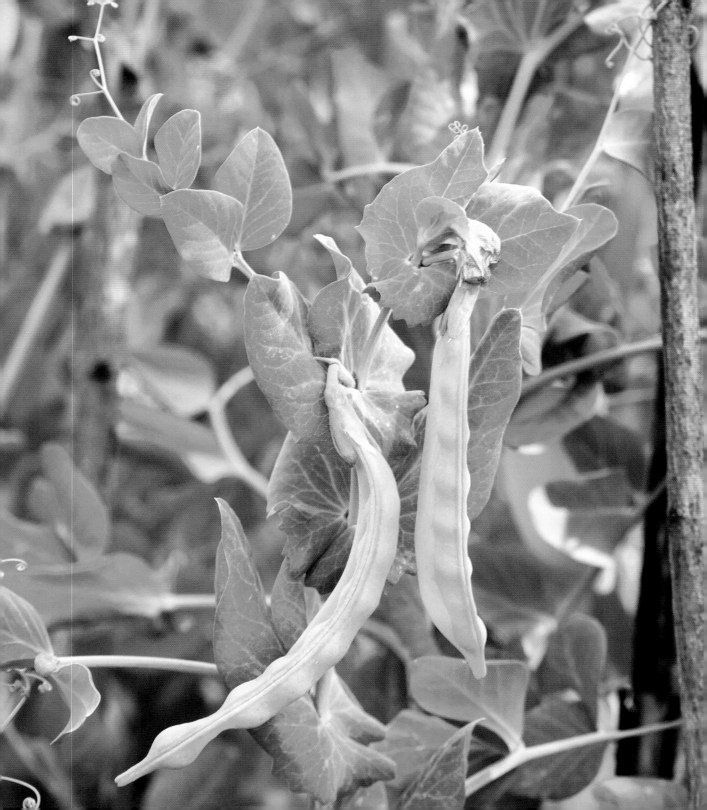

REMEMBER THAT LEGUMES ARE GOOD NOT ONLY IN TRADITIONAL DISHES, BUT ADDED TO SMOOTHIES, SOUPS, AND BREADS, TOO.

and ends up instead in the large intestine where the nutrients ferment with help of the intestinal bacteria. As a result you produce gas, which is not always comfortable or pleasant. It is proof, though, that the blood sugar is being absorbed as slowly as possible.

A study done with common beans showed that their anti-nutrients not only lowered the blood sugar response after a meal, but also increased feelings of satiety. A very interesting observation was that ghrelin levels decreased after eating beans, which should lead to fewer sugar cravings.

FIND THE BALANCE

Legumes are cheap and nutritious food, two of the many reasons you should make them a regular staple of your diet. However, it's important that you find your individual level of tolerance in order to reap their benefit while avoiding problems with gastric distress, swelling, and gas.

It's assumed that the body gets used to legumes, as some of the effect is due to their high fiber content. The body is adaptable, so the best way to get used to them is to eat a few legumes every day. A few tablespoons of hummus or a side of black beans at dinner is enough to impart their health effects, with very little gas. Increase the amount gradually, and remember that canned legumes are more digestible than the dry ones you prepare from scratch. If you do decide to start with dried beans, using a pressure cooker is a great help: cooking legumes this way makes food break down more readily and thus becomes much more digestible.

Remember that legumes are tasty not only in traditional dishes, but added to smoothies, soups, and breads, too. Add mashed beans to the eggs of your omelet, or enjoy a glass of wine with a side of edamame (soy beans) to snack on.

The body tends to tolerate lentils better than peas, which in turn are easier on the digestion than beans. Explore a variety of legumes to find your level of tolerance, and your blood sugar balance will surely benefit.

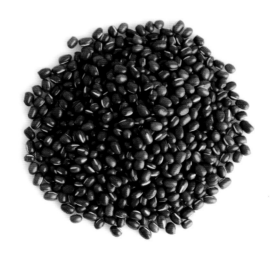

36

Sugar and Inflammation

INFLAMMATION—A SURE ROAD TO DISEASE

We've all experienced inflammation from time to time. Sore joints and muscles, stomach- and headaches are among its usual manifestations. The word *inflammo* is Latin and means, roughly speaking, "I'm burning." In many cases this is an apt description of what is happening.

Inflammation can also have less acutely painful expressions like acne, hay fever, eczema, and dementia. The fact is, inflammation is behind many serious illnesses such as edentulism (tooth loss), cardiovascular disease, cancer, and autoimmune diseases. Among the latter you can include rheumatism, ulcerous colitis, Crohn's disease, type 1 diabetes, and MS (multiple sclerosis).

Sometimes inflammation affects specific organs, such as the prostate or the kidneys, and often increases the risk for complications and decreased functioning of the organs in question.

As you've probably figured out, too much inflammation is something we want to avoid.

However, it's necessary in many ways—we still need it to repair microscopic damage in our blood vessels. Workout soreness is also, after all, self-inflicted inflammation that leads to positive results such as an increase in muscle mass and strength.

Inflammation is also the body's own defense against viruses, poisons, and bacteria, which is not to be confused with infection. Infections are caused by microorganisms, include the production of pus, and are often painful. That said, prolonged infections can result in inflammation, and because of this it's important for the body to sustain a balance between pro-inflammatory and anti-inflammatory processes.

A PRO-INFLAMMATORY PRODUCT

One of the most damaging effects of high sugar intake is due to sugar's pro-inflammatory properties. Much research has shown that the more sugar one consumes, the greater the likelihood of inflammation, and the more dangerous sugar is to eat.

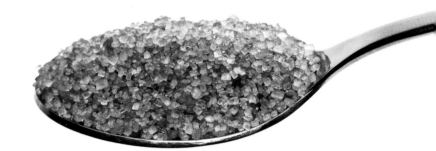

Sugar is, chemically, pure carbohydrates, and lacks all anti-inflammatory substances such as flavonoids, prebiotics (fibers that promote the growth of beneficial bacteria), salicylates, resveratrol, fatty acids, probiotics (beneficial bacteria), and many others that exist in natural foods.

It also seems that sugar encourages the growth of pro-inflammatory bacteria in the gut. Much research supports this, and even that a diet rich in fats does the same **(107)**.

Another plausible explanation for sugar's pro-inflammatory properties is that it makes you gain weight. Adipose tissue is a powerful producer of various pro-inflammatory molecules, so logically, the higher your weight, the more inflammation is likely to be present.

Inflammation can also come from reactions we have in response to AGEs, which are brought about when heat reacts upon sugar—such as in cookies, toffee, caramel, pancakes, etc. **(101)**.

Weight reduction is a natural outcome of a sugar-free life, and therefore automatically leads to less inflammation.

SUGAR CREATES INFLAMMATION

A study of 4,800 children between the ages of 3 and 11 years showed that high consumption of soda didn't just increase bad cholesterol (LDL) but also CRP **(108)**.

CRP is the acronym for C-reactive protein and is a marker of inflammation.

In other words, even young, healthy individuals incur damage caused by sugar consumption.

Another study showed that food with a low glycemic index—in other words, a sugar-free diet—decreased the incidence of acne considerably, and even reduced other inflammation-inducing substances in the body **(109)**.

In a study of middle-aged subjects (average age 49 years) it was shown that sugar consumption was connected to the risk of dying from an inflammation-caused illness **(110)**.

37

The Magic of Spices

CINNAMON AND BLOOD SUGAR

Researchers have long attempted to find a way to reduce blood sugar response after a meal, and it turns out that one of the tastiest and simplest ways to do so is to eat spices. Focus has been mostly on cinnamon because it has shown itself to be extremely valuable—one way being by lowering blood sugar response in both overweight people as well as those of healthy weight.

In one study, participants were given 6 grams (0.21 ounce) of ground cinnamon to eat with 50 grams (2 ounces) of carbohydrates in the form of breakfast cereal flakes. Those who ate cinnamon with their meal experienced a significantly lower blood sugar level 15, 30, 45, and 60 minutes after ingesting the meal, compared to the participants who did not have cinnamon [111].

The reason cinnamon is so beneficial is that its water-soluble antioxidants (called polyphenols) have an insulin-like effect on muscles and the liver. This makes it unnecessary for the body to use a lot of insulin to balance the blood sugar, which is preferable since too much insulin can cause weight gain, type 2 diabetes, cardiovascular disease, and a faster growth of cancer cells.

Another study showed that 1 gram (0.03 ounce) of cinnamon isn't enough to decrease the insulin response, while 3 grams (0.11 ounce) were plenty [112]. Several other studies have shown similar results. Thus, cinnamon is beneficial to blood sugar [113, 114, 115] and therefore to your health. 2 to 6 grams (0.07–0.21 ounce) taken daily, depending on your need, should be a sufficient dose.

THE BENEFITS OF FENUGREEK

Indian and Thai dishes often use fenugreek in their curry mixes. The spice has shown, much like cinnamon, to have advantageous properties for blood sugar control. It also appears to strengthen the nervous system, reduce blood lipids, and have calming as well as antibacterial properties [116].

Other ascribed attributes include alleviating migraines, improving memory, and blocking the development of cancer **(116)**.

Animal research has shown that extract of fenugreek can reverse pathological changes (i.e., fatty degeneration) in the liver, pancreas, heart, and kidneys **(117)**. It can allegedly stimulate regeneration of beta cells in the pancreas, which would in theory increase the body's ability to produce insulin if it is hampered **(116)**.

Fenugreek has several biologically active ingredients, the most studied of which is trigonelline, an alkaloid that fenugreek has in large amounts.

Follow my advice and add more curry to your food! Then you'll also get turmeric, which offers even more benefits for your health.

TURMERIC PROMOTES BETTER INSULIN SENSITIVITY

Curry's yellow color comes from turmeric, a rather mild spice with a strong anti-inflammatory effect. Through animal studies it has also shown to possibly contain blood sugar balancing properties.

Diabetic rats that were fed turmeric in their yogurt became healthier, showing better blood sugar balance than animals that were not given the spiced yogurt **(118)**. Muscles' insulin sensitivity seems to be improved by eating turmeric **(119)**, which is a highly desirable effect. Then carbohydrates entering the muscles are more likely to be burned as fuel, instead of being routed to the fat cells to be stored as fat.

Try spicing up your food—it's one of the simplest ways to improve your blood sugar balance.

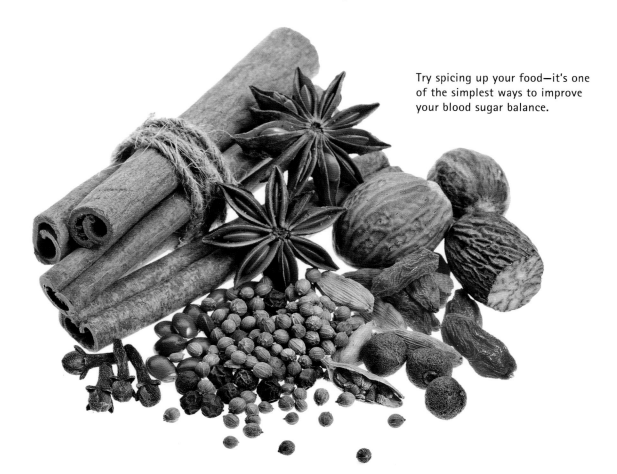

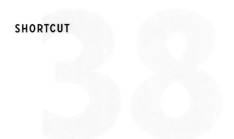

Drink Coffee and Tea

BALANCED BLOOD SUGAR WITH COFFEE AND TEA

It's important that blood sugar not be too elevated. It's damaging to your health, in addition to making you feel tired and out of sorts. Coffee exerts a very good influence on blood sugar balance because it helps cells process glucose.

Why this happens is not quite clear, but it might be due to coffee's high content of natural antioxidants, which protect the insulin receptors from oxidative stress and keep insulin sensitivity intact.

Keep in mind that it's not the caffeine per say that's good for your blood sugar—quite the contrary. If you drink too many colas or energy drinks (Red Bull, for example) you'll get pure caffeine but no antioxidants, and the caffeine will then lower your insulin sensitivity.

200 milligrams of caffeine is enough to see an 18 percent lowering of insulin sensitivity and a 19 percent increase in blood sugar **(120)**. In the long run, this increases your risk for type 2 diabetes.

One reason caffeine has this effect is that it releases free fatty acids from the fat cells, as this is nature's way of responding to food that is low in carbohydrates but rich in fat. The body wants to save all the important glucose for the brain and not divert it to the muscles, and the only way to accomplish this is by lowering insulin sensitivity. The problem is that this is a false alarm, because there is already plenty of glucose, so much so that it eventually becomes harmful.

If for any reason you need a shot of pure caffeine, make sure to use up lots of free fatty acids. How do you do this? The most effective way is, without a doubt, to move your body. Working muscles take up free fatty acids and use them as fuel, so it's possible that exercise actively reduces the harm caused by caffeine.

END YOUR MEAL WITH A CUP OF COFFEE

Chlorogenic acid is a component in coffee, and tea has high levels of the antioxidant EGCG (epigallocatechin gallate).

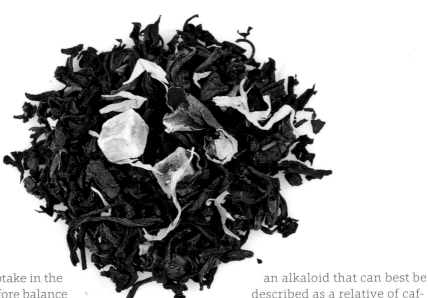

Both inhibit glucose uptake in the small intestine and therefore balance the blood sugar **(121)**. Coffee and tea are strongly associated with a decreased risk of type 2 diabetes **(122, 123)**, the main reason being possibly that they act as inhibitors, which is a good enough reason to end your meal with a coffee and not worry that any nutrients will be lost.

When I'm on a lecture tour, the question of how healthy coffee and tea are comes up often; there seems to be a common belief that they'll lower the uptake of vitamins and minerals. There exists no research indicating that anyone has suffered nutritional deficiency due to drinking coffee or tea with food. In fact, you ought to consider these beverages as welcome additions to your meal because of the abundance of antioxidants included in them.

Coffee contains, aside from chlorogenic acid, an enormously rich cocktail of chemical substances that positively impact health in many different ways.

One such substance that inhibits the uptake of glucose in the gut is trigonelline, which is an alkaloid that can best be described as a relative of caffeine, as it imparts beneficial yet completely different effects **(124)**.

TEA DRINKING IS SIMILAR TO A SMALL WORKOUT

When you engage in exercise, your blood sugar decreases because muscles need energy, and they'll use what's readily available to them. A working muscle makes the protein GLUT-4, which in turn makes the muscle cells permeable and allows the blood sugar to enter into the muscles instead of swimming around in the blood.

An interesting observation is that tea—either green or black—seems to have a similar effect to sustained physical activity: it increases the GLUT-4 in the muscles and balances the blood sugar **(125)**. Red tea is the exception, however, because it's not produced from the same plant as the other types of tea. We don't know very much about red tea yet, except that it's good for you due to its high concentration of antioxidants.

39

Fermented and Sour Foods

FERMENTED AND SOUR FOODS ARE GOOD FOR BLOOD SUGAR

We've been aware for a long time that fermented foods lower blood sugar levels. Sour ingredients and nutrients have low GI value and actively lower the pH of food, which in turn tells the stomach to hang on to the food a bit longer.

Some people will drink a glass of water in which they've added a teaspoon of apple cider vinegar before their meal in an effort to prevent possible blood sugar spikes, but that seems a tad excessive. Much simpler—and more appetizing—is to use lemon, vinegar, lime, or yogurt to season the foods you're cooking. You can even include fermented milk, sauerkraut, or sour berries and fruit to reach the same effect.

I like to drink lemon water, and I mix vinegar into my salad dressing, so tart and sour foods taste perfectly normal to me. I love to pour dressing over the warm rice, quinoa, or oat kernels I'm preparing for dinner. It adds flavor and nourishment, and I make my favorite vinaigrette from scratch with olive oil and red wine vinegar.

Red wine vinegar contains quite a few antioxidants, which unfortunately cannot be said for white wine vinegar. Balsamic vinegar has been aged, and therefore contains AGE—the damaged nutrients that increase inflammation in the body—so I can't recommend eating dishes that count it among its ingredients. Rice vinegar, on the other hand, is a good alternative.

Sourdough brings down blood sugar levels due to the acidity that builds up in the dough when the yeast is at work. Wine contains acidity, which might be a contributing factor to its ability to lower blood sugar response after a meal. The alcohol itself might be instrumental to the blood sugar response as much as the antioxidants.

LACTO-FERMENTED VEGETABLES

A few years ago there were hardly any lacto-fermented vegetables—especially non pasteurized ones—to be had in the Swedish

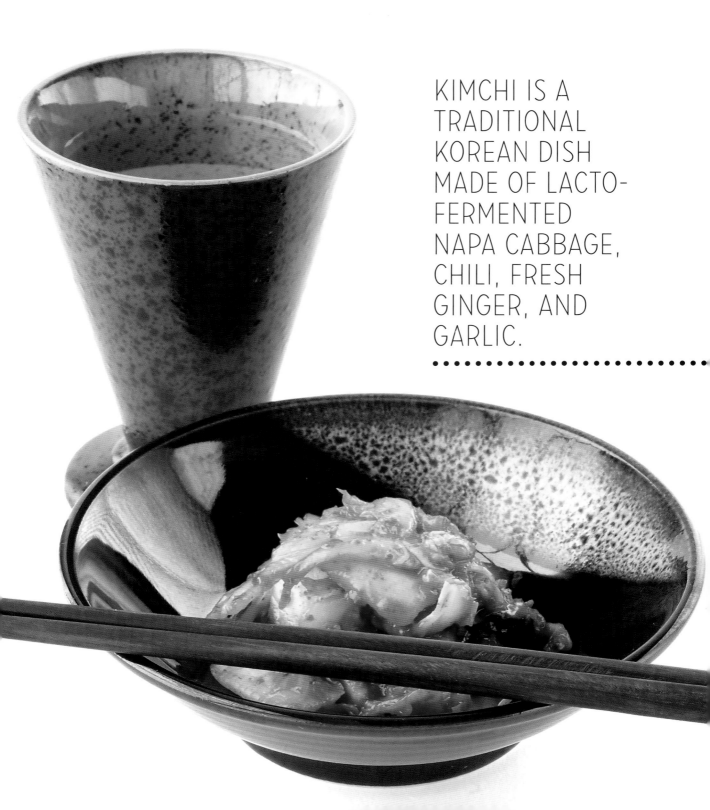

KIMCHI IS A TRADITIONAL KOREAN DISH MADE OF LACTO-FERMENTED NAPA CABBAGE, CHILI, FRESH GINGER, AND GARLIC.

grocery stores. During pasteurization, a container of food is heated, and the bacteria that could otherwise grow within and become a health hazard are killed; sadly, this process also kills the culture of lactobacillus that is so good for your body.

For instance, when you eat sauerkraut, lactobacillus (also referred to as acidofila) start to colonize in your mouth, which freshens the breath and protects against tooth decay. They proceed down to the stomach where lactobacillus can thrive, as they prefer an acidic environment. There, they guard against bacteria such as Heliobacter pylori, which otherwise might cause stomach ulcers.

Lactobacillus continues down into the small intestine, where they support normal peristalsis, optimize nutrient uptake, and strengthen the immune system.

The last way station is the large intestine, where they exist in large amounts and keep disease-causing bacteria and other microorganisms at bay.

In addition, lactobacillus has a positive effect on the brain, since the gut and the brain are in constant communication. Research has shown that healthy intestinal flora produces lower levels of stress hormones in the blood. When you eat lactobacillus, the GI value of the meal decreases. A lower pH means more acidity, and as we know, this leads to slower emptying of the stomach contents and a lower blood sugar response.

I heartily recommend adding more lacto-fermented vegetables to your dinner plate. My personal favorite is the Korean cabbage dish called kimchi. It's made from Napa cabbage that has been lacto-fermented together with chili, fresh ginger, and garlic. It's delicate, it evens out the blood sugar, and is terrifically wholesome!

PAULÚN'S SALAD DRESSING
Blend together 1 tablespoon red wine vinegar, 4 tablespoons extra-virgin olive oil, and 1 crushed garlic clove. Season with herb salt. and salt to taste.
This is good on salads as well as added to warm rice or quinoa.

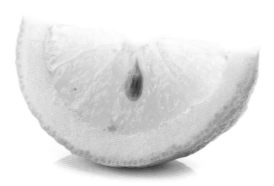

40

Vitamin D Balances Blood Sugar

VITAMIN D'S MANY FUNCTIONS

In the last few years vitamin D's importance has sparked lively debate in health newsletters and Internet forums. It has proven to be a vitamin that has many functions in the body, one of which being to help build bone matter. It helps the body regulate blood levels of calcium and phosphorus in a way that optimizes the re-mineralization of the skeleton.

There are also many indications that vitamin D acts on the body's neurological processes, and that a lack of this nutrient increases the risk of Parkinson's disease, multiple sclerosis, and depression. In addition, a deficiency might negatively impact the immune system and raise the risk of cancer and cardiovascular disease.

Vitamin D is also deemed necessary for a safe and healthy pregnancy, especially since a woman's immune system must be strong yet nurturing enough to carry a fetus to term. Studies have shown that mortality is inversely correlated to the level of vitamin D

VITAMIN D AND YOUR BLOOD SUGAR

Several studies have shown that low levels of vitamin D increase the risk of developing type 2 diabetes (126,127).

As type 2 diabetes can be described as a state of high insulin insensitivity, this marks it as an extreme condition within a broad spectrum. You don't need to be clinically diagnosed with type 2 diabetes to suffer from depressed insulin sensitivity, which manifests itself through fatigue, weight gain, elevated blood pressure, and increased appetite.

We can therefore consider vitamin D a potent asset in balancing blood sugar, which should be used early on as a preventative measure against type 2 diabetes.

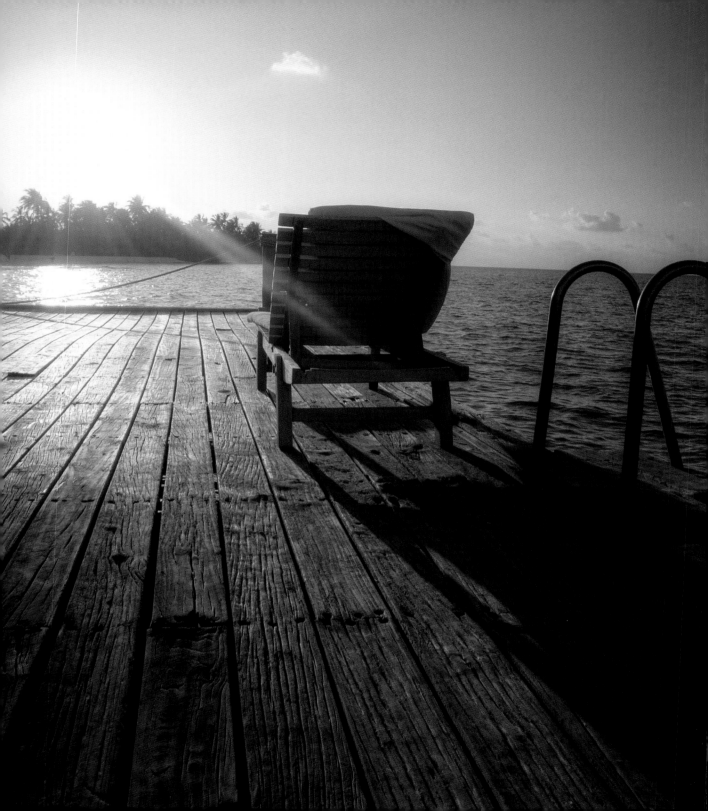

in the blood—the less vitamin D, the higher the risk of dying prematurely.

Considering all its other plentiful benefits, it shouldn't be surprising then that vitamin D is also helpful in regulating blood sugar.

Research has also shown that supplementation of vitamin D during pregnancy lessens the risk of developing gestational diabetes (128), which is unhealthy for both the mother and the fetus. So if having a healthy level of vitamin D is one of your best strategies for blood sugar control, how do you achieve it?

VITAMIN D FROM FOOD AND SUN

By definition, a vitamin is something that needs to be supplied to the body through food, and therefore vitamin D is not, strictly speaking, a vitamin, as it is made when ultraviolet (UV) light shines on the skin.

If you sunbathe in the summer clad only in a swimsuit, your body will produce 10,000 to 20,000 IUs (international units) of vitamin D in half an hour. If you slather on a sunscreen of SPF 8, the vitamin D production plummets by 95% (129)!

My own strategy is to more or less skip using sunscreen, and instead stay in the shadow when the sun is too strong.

Wearing clothes made from thin cotton fabric offers good protection against sunburn, while still enabling you to reap the benefit of the sun's vitamin D producing effect. Then you'll also avoid using sunscreens, some of which might possibly be injurious to your health.

In the wintertime, however, even on a bright sunny day, there is not enough natural light for this process to take place. For this reason, to be on the safe side, we need to ensure that our bodies get vitamin D

VITAMIN D CONTENT IN FISH

120 grams (4¼ ounces)—one serving—contains this much Vitamin D:

Rainbow Trout	16.3 micrograms
Salmon	15 micrograms
Herring	14.4 micrograms
Baltic Herring	11 micrograms
Mackerel	4.7 micrograms
Cod	1.2 micrograms
Northern Pike	1 microgram
Perch	1 microgram

through food and supplements. If you live at northern latitudes and you are in a position to do so, it's a good idea to take a vacation in a sunny destination to make up for the seasonal lack of daylight hours. This is especially important if you suffer from type 2 diabetes or are pre diabetic.

Also, focus on eating the following foods if you want to get enough Vitamin D through food: fatty fish, egg yolks, full-fat dairy, and liver. Eels hold the record for vitamin D content, but the species is threatened with extinction, making it ecologically unsound to eat, unless you can find a source of farmed eel.

Otherwise, vitamin D supplements are a good way to go, especially during the shorter days of the year.

41

The Beneficial Whole Grain

RESISTANCE AND COMPLETE NUTRITION

Our forefathers ate food that contained different kinds of whole grains. Think of seeds and corn growing wild. If you pick up a few grains from, say, a field of oats, and chew them, you'll see that they put up quite a lot of resistance; it'll be obvious when you swallow them that the kernels have remained pretty much intact. They've only flattened a bit, and this means that they're sending a signal to the stomach to take its time digesting, so the stomach empties slower, the way it should. In earlier times, most foods were very rough and chewy, and it's not until the last few centuries that it has, on the whole, become possible to consume completely processed and refined foods such as sugars, oils, cooking fats, dehydrated mixes, starches, and the like.

Whole grains have had their hard outer shell removed, but the nutritious inner shell remains intact. They contain large amounts of nutrients, only a few of which have been mapped, such as vitamins, minerals, and antioxidants, but there are certainly more types that are beneficial for us.

Research shows that whole grain products are linked to better insulin sensitivity and lower blood sugar response (130). In one study, participants (who were all cardiovascular patients) were given a daily serving of whole grain products for sixteen weeks. During that time their blood sugar levels decreased by 24 percent, and their insulin levels went down by 14 percent (131). Their antioxidant status improved as well, leading to the conclusion that you should opt to eat whole grains whenever possible.

HOW TO USE GRAINS AND WHOLEMEAL

Make sure the flour you use when you cook or bake from scratch is whole meal. It's simple and very easy to get used to the taste. You can even get your carbohydrates from whole grains such as brown rice and whole wheat pasta.

There are also a number of other whole grain products—often overlooked—such

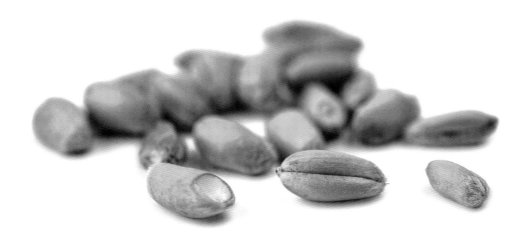

as corn, oat kernels, rolled oats, rye, shredded wheat, and quinoa, which all have their nutritious inner shell intact (this excludes couscous). Less commonly used grains such as spelt, amaranth, kamut wheat, teff, buckwheat, and farro are also very healthy.

When you shop at the grocery store, always choose products containing large amounts of whole grains. The GI Index is not always low but the nutritional value is always high, so overall the effect on the blood sugar is beneficial. Unsurprisingly, it has been shown that a high consumption of whole grain products lowers the risk for type 2 diabetes **(132)**.

WHAT IS THE DIFFERENCE BETWEEN WHOLE GRAINS AND REFINED PRODUCTS?

Whole grains contain fewer carbohydrates and more protein, as well as more fiber, than products based on the content of the shelled kernel. This translates to fewer calories per 100 grams (or 3½ ounces) of food. Whole grains also have lesser-known substances like arabinoxylans, a special kind of fiber with different phenolic acids. These nutrients are antioxidants, and are natural fungus fighters. An exciting phenolic lipid called alkylresorcinol also appears to have cancer-inhibiting properties.

Whole grain products may also contain substances such as tocols and phytosterols. Tocols are strong antioxidants that are commonly found in black, unprocessed rice. Phytosterols exist in all kinds of whole grain products, and have a lowering effect on blood lipids **(133)**. A large investigation comparing eighteen different study results showed that eating a serving of whole grains decreased inflammation in the body by a significant amount. The marker of inflammation CRP (C-reactive protein) was measured and it decreased by 7 percent with each serving of whole grain consumed **(134)**.

42

Fiber and Blood Sugar

SOLUBLE AND INSOLUBLE FIBER

Fiber is defined as the part of our food that cannot be absorbed by the blood and stays in the intestine. It might be in the form of insoluble fiber, which is metabolically inert and not used by the flora in the large intestine. It's used basically as added bulk, tasked to help move things along by insuring proper peristalsis.

Certain insoluble fiber does ferment in the gut with the help of bacteria, and gas is created when the fiber is broken down into short fatty acids that you can then absorb. You'll get a positive, so-called prebiotic effect on the intestinal flora from this process, which is one of the big bonuses from eating fiber. Fiber fermentation itself actually provides some energy, contrary to what was previously thought.

Soluble fiber, also called water-soluble fiber, is more interesting from a blood sugar perspective, as it mixes with water and turns into gel. (Try soaking a few tablespoons of crushed flaxseeds and you'll see what I mean.) This fiber also has a good prebiotic effect, but most important, it slows down digestion, which leads

to more balanced blood sugar. Much suggests that water-soluble fiber provides satiety in the same way as fat with the help of the intestinal hormone CCK (cholecystokinin) **(135)**.

BEST SOURCES OF FIBER

Beans, lentils, and peas are tremendous sources of water-soluble fiber, and they are also instrumental in slowing blood sugar increases thanks to their antioxidant content. A few tablespoons of legumes with a meal will decrease the blood sugar load of the entire meal.

We've already mentioned nuts and seeds in another part of the book, and yet we bring them up again here because their benefit to blood sugar levels is due to their high content of water-soluble fiber.

Fruits and berries are great providers of water-soluble fiber: plums, ripe bananas, apples, and pears are especially good sources. Broccoli, carrots, and sweet potatoes are also recommended for their high fiber content.

It's not by chance that fruit and vegetables have been chosen to be the poster children in the promotion of wholesome, healthy food.

Many industrially manufactured foods such as breakfast cereal, bread, and biscuits also contain a wide variety of fiber. Oligo-fructose, a subgroup of inulin, is especially beneficial as a prebiotic fiber that stimulates the growth of lactobacillus and bifido-bacteria. When these bacteria break down inulin, the result is short fatty acid chains and increased uptake of minerals like calcium and magnesium.

It's a good idea to occasionally take a supplement containing water-soluble fiber if your diet is generally poor and lacking in naturally fiber- rich foods. Products such as guar gum and glucomannan have both proven to work by providing satiety and by balancing blood sugar.

Psyllium and flaxseed are also well known for their high content of water-soluble fiber—flaxseed especially since it's often a topic of research. In a study involving type 2 diabetic participants, it was shown that taking 10 grams (0.35 ounce) of round flaxseed per day over the course of a month lowered blood sugar by almost 20 percent **(136)**! Glycated hemoglobin decreased by 15 percent, which proves that flaxseed offers very good protection against harmful blood sugar levels. It's no surprise then that a higher intake of fiber has generally shown to increase life span in humans **(137)**.

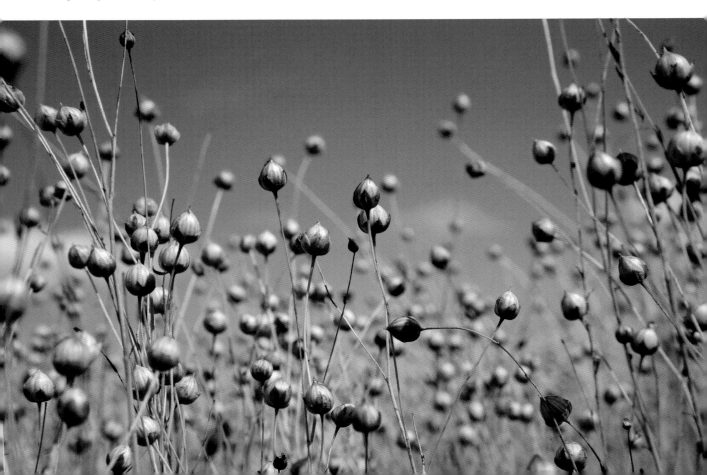

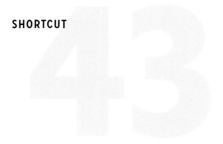

ALA (Alpha-Lipoic Acid) for Better Blood Sugar

A SUPER STRONG ANTIOXIDANT

Alpha-ipoic acid, thioctic acid, and ALA are three of many scientific names given to the same antioxidant. This substance has gotten a lot of attention as it has shown to have beneficial health effects on diseases such as multiple sclerosis, age-related cognitive problems, and cardiovascular disease.

The reason I mention ALA here is that it supposedly increases insulin sensitivity in people with type 1 diabetes. In Germany it has been used for decades, and with great success, in the treatment of type 1 diabetes. We also know that ALA improves insulin sensitivity for those with type 2 diabetes (138). In animal research, ALA has prevented the development of fatty liver and other pathological changes in the liver brought on by high fructose intake (139).

By what exact mechanism ALA works is not quite clear, but it's likely due to its strong antioxidant effect. It might also have a role in protecting the insulin receptors against oxidative stress and keeping them functional. Since high blood sugar levels are known to increase free radicals and damage those receptors, this antioxidant has important ramifications.

ALA is also interesting in that it seems to charge and restore other antioxidants, like vitamin C, that have been damaged by free radicals.

WHERE DO WE FIND ALA?

ALA is commonly found in green leafy vegetables and tomatoes. Tomato juice and tomato purée are good examples because they're readily absorbed. I'm aware that a lot of research has been done on fermented tomato juice as a way to control blood sugar, and it seems to work well—you not only get ALA and other antioxidants, but also see an improvement in intestinal flora.

Even broccoli is a good source of ALA. Perhaps the high content of this acid in vegetables is one more reason (along with their low carbohydrates, high water, and high fiber content) they're so beneficial for blood sugar balance.

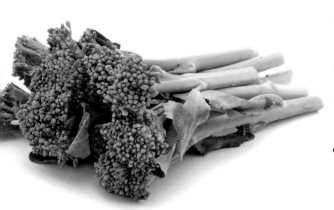

LIPOIC ACID SEEMS TO RESTORE ANTIOXIDANTS THAT HAVE BEEN DAMAGED BY FREE RADICALS.

ALA is found in offal such as liver, heart, and kidney; however, few of these foods are regularly eaten in most parts of the world, so we don't consider them a significant source.

ALA is an endogenous substance, as the human body produces some by itself. Different health crises can hamper its production, however, and it may prove difficult for people whose level of ALA has been depleted from illness to replenish enough of it through food alone. If this is the case, then it's appropriate to take it as a supplement.

ALA SUPPLEMENTATION

I would not hesitate to take an ALA supplement if I were diagnosed with a diabetic condition. It's effective, reasonably priced, and appears to have no negative side effects.

Research shows that taking a daily dose of ALA—between 300 to 600 milligrams—is not only harmless, but can be beneficial **(140)**. For example, test subjects experienced less nerve damage from their illness, and found it easier to control pain, when they took ALA. Individuals with type 2 diabetes tend to suffer from cardiovascular disease at a higher rate than healthy people, and ALA is considered a helpful tool for limiting this risk **(141)**.

The amount of ALA to use as a preventative measure is a topic of debate in the scientific community. Nevertheless, higher doses of ALA don't appear to bring on any adverse effects. Instead, improvement in insulin sensitivity has been directly linked to ALA when the following dosages were compared: 300, 600, 900, and 1,200 milligrams daily **(142)**. There are no observational studies recording the effect of doses larger than 1 gram per day over several years, so there's always a risk that mega doses might give rise to unwanted side effects. However, since diabetes has already been established as a harmful disease that's hard to control, prescribing large doses might at some point be justified.

44

Chromium and Blood Sugar

WHAT IS CHROMIUM'S ROLE?

There are a few substances that are absolutely essential for blood sugar control in the body, and chromium and ALA (alpha-lipoic acid) are two of them. Researchers have known since the 1980s that a lack of chromium can lead to symptoms similar to those of type 2 diabetes.

Chromium's role was unclear for a long time, until it was discovered that as part of the enigmatically named GTF (glucose tolerance factor) its central function is to bind insulin to its receptors.

Keep in mind that the type of chromium normally found in food is trivalent (chromium 3+) and biologically active; this should not be confused with hexavalent chromium (chromium 6+), which is extremely poisonous and has a place on the MSDS (Material Safety Data Sheet), a document that lists risks for work environments such as manufacturing plants and factories. That said, even trivalent chromium can be consumed in excess, especially if you take too many supplements.

When chromium became a popular dietary supplement in the 1980s, it could be found in a multitude of powders and capsules marketed for weight gain (for improved nutritional uptake) or weight loss (to lessen sugar cravings and increase fat burning). This became a cause for concern to nutritional experts, since overenthusiastic supplement users sometimes ingested 5 to 10 times the recommended—and safe—dose of chromium.

DO I NEED DIETARY SUPPLEMENTS?

You don't need to take a supplement containing chromium if you're healthy, but if your insulin sensitivity is lowered, then it might be something worth trying. The cost of chromium supplements is negligible, and they're safe as long as you follow the recommended dosage.

According to the American Diabetics Association (2012), 29.1 million Americans, or 9.3 percent of the population, had diabetes, and of that number, 8.1 million were undiagnosed. These individuals really do have a reason to try chromium. The dosage should be kept to a daily 200 micrograms—a tiny amount. We're talking about 200 millionths of a gram! It wouldn't be visible to the naked eye if you put it in the palm of your hand.

If you don't suffer from type 2 diabetes and you're not pre diabetic, you'll have nothing to gain from taking chromium supplements. In fact, research has shown that healthy individuals who ingested high doses of chromium—in this particular study it amounted to 1,000 micrograms daily over 16 days—actually ended up with lowered insulin sensitivity (143).

WHERE DO I FIND CHROMIUM?

It's easy to get enough chromium through a nutritious and balanced diet. That way it's unlikely that you'll overdose and inadvertently lower your insulin sensitivity. The very best source for dietary chromium is brewer's yeast, but it's hardly a feature on many daily menus unless you take it as a supplement. However, years ago it was a common ingredient in vitamin B complex.

Some common everyday foods that contain chromium are eggs, red meat, liver, chicken, oysters, spinach, bananas, green peppers, wheat germ, and apples. On page 105 you read about hazelnuts (filberts) and their chromium content. You'll also find it in butter, black peppercorns, and molasses. You shouldn't need to worry about your level of chromium, as your daily intake of food more than likely fulfills your daily requirement; regardless, it's good to know where to find it.

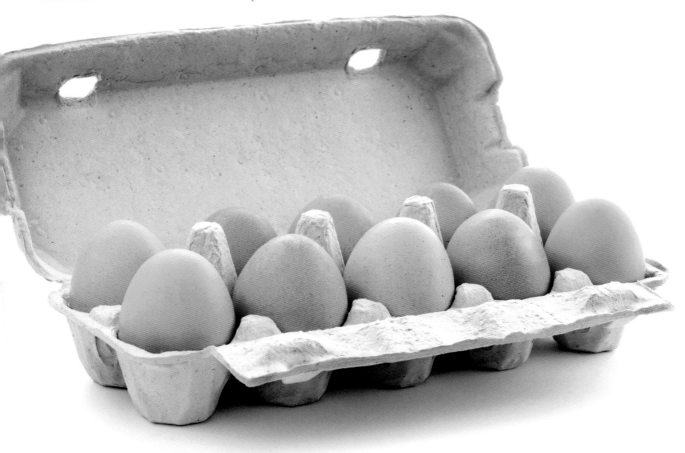

45

Eat Fish

THE WONDER PROTEIN

We've known for a long time now that fish is good for our health in many ways. What many people may not be aware of, however, is that fish is one of the best sources of protein to keep the body's blood sugar in check. While other fatty meats lower insulin sensitivity, fish increases it due to some unique properties of its protein and its fat.

While all proteins slow down the emptying of the stomach, fish protein goes one further: it breaks down into smaller peptides (protein stumps) that are absorbed into the bloodstream and improve insulin sensitivity **(144)**. As fish itself is very rich in protein, one benefits from other important advantages of eating protein, notably increased satiety and stabilized blood sugar.

OMEGA-3 GIVES BALANCED BLOOD SUGAR

Omega-3 fatty acids are found in crops as ALA (alpha-lipoic acid), and in fish and seafood as DHA (docosahexaenoic acid), EPA (ecosapentaenoic acid), and DPA (docosapentaenoic acid). Fish contains mostly DHA and EPA, and the fattier the fish, the higher the content of these fatty acids. DHA and EPA are highly polyunsaturated, which means they are of low viscosity. It's possible to see this with the naked eye if you keep a bottle of fish oil in the fridge: the oil will remain liquid even when it's cold, while butter, which consists of mostly saturated fat, will become a solid block when chilled. This is due to the fats' saturation level, and the least saturated fats are the healthier, liquid omega-3 fatty acids. They only solidify at extremely low temperatures, and because of this property they keep our cell membranes soft, which in turn improves our sensitivity to insulin and our blood sugar control.

LOADED WITH VITAMIN D

Very few foods are as loaded with vitamin D as fish. You can read more about this on page 131. Fatty fish in particular, such as herring, salmon, char, eel, Baltic herring, and mackerel, are exceptional in vitamin D content.

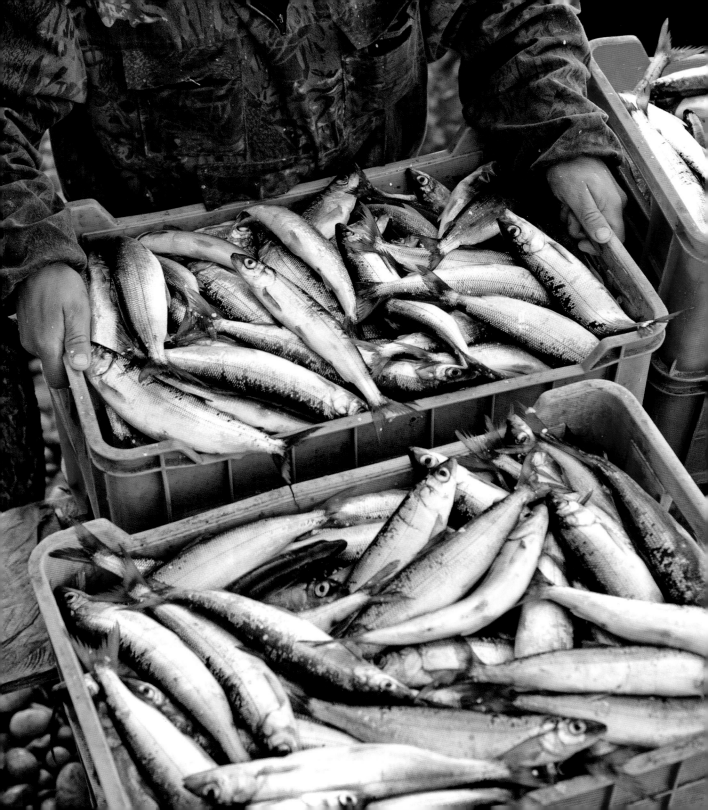

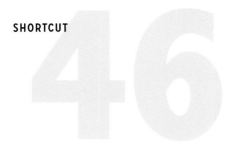

Gluten-free Done Correctly

EAT WHOLESOME FOOD EVEN IF YOU MUST AVOID GLUTEN

There are many who don't feel well after they've eaten something containing gluten, which is a form of protein found in wheat, barley, and rye.

Biologists have a theory as to why this happens: part of gluten's defense function in cereals is to damage the intestine of the creature wanting to eat it. However, since the epithelial cells inside the small intestine are replaced very quickly (they replenish themselves approximately every 48 hours), most of us manage to eat gluten without any ill effects.

For any number of reasons, some people develop intolerance or an allergy of varying degrees of severity to gluten, and this can cause a slew of symptoms.

The most familiar manifestation of these adverse reactions is celiac disease, which is caused by an overly sensitive small intestine that reacts to even the smallest gluten molecule.

The classic symptoms of celiac disease are intense stomach pains, bloody stool, and diarrhea, which in the long run can lead to malnutrition and weight loss. It's reasonably easy to diagnose celiac disease, but lately we've seen other types of flare-ups that are more or less caused by the consumption of gluten.

In magazines and on websites devoted to diet and health, there are speculations that gluten is far more problematic than first thought. It is posited that as gluten damages the intestine, the body goes one further and produces antibodies against it.

Even if it doesn't lead to celiac disease, gluten sensitivity can cause eczema, migraine, fatigue, weight gain, aching joints, and gastric distress. As it allegedly damages the intestine, even illnesses such Crohn's disease and ulcerous colitis are connected to excess gluten consumption. Injury to the intestine can leak undigested food molecules into the bloodstream, and this alone can bring on allergies or cause autoimmune diseases such as type 1 diabetes and rheumatism.

IS GLUTEN DANGEROUS?

It's starting to sound as though gluten might be poisonous to us all, but that is far from true.

Only when it causes a negative reaction does it need to be avoided. If you suffer no ill effects from gluten, then it should pose no threat to you if it's part of wholesome foods like rye flakes, spelt, whole-wheat flour, and pearl barley.

Refined white flour, on the other hand, should be avoided unless it can be eaten in tandem with some other, more nutritious food. Whole-wheat bread and pasta, for example, have some refined white flour blended in, yet can still be considered healthy food. What is unhealthy, however, is eating gluten despite being intolerant of it, as the consequence could be increased inflammation in the body, as well as an increased risk of developing serious diseases like cancer and cardiovascular disease.

So if you don't suffer from any symptoms of gluten intolerance, you have nothing to worry about. If you suspect that you might be sensitive to it—if you experience unexplained fatigue for instance, or if you develop eczema—it would be a smart move to set gluten aside for a couple weeks to see if your health improves. If nothing changes, gluten might not be the culprit.

GLUTEN-FREE THE CORRECT WAY

If you choose to follow a gluten-free diet—whether as a short stint or over a long period of time—you should choose naturally gluten-free alternatives. Manufactured products like gluten-free breads or pastas are often extremely unhealthy, as they replace wheat flour with different kinds of starches such as refined wheat starch, cornstarch, or rice starch, which are all comparable to pure fructose. They're empty calories that elevate blood sugar in an instant, so they should be avoided at all costs. It's difficult to imagine anything worse in terms of nutrition than those products.

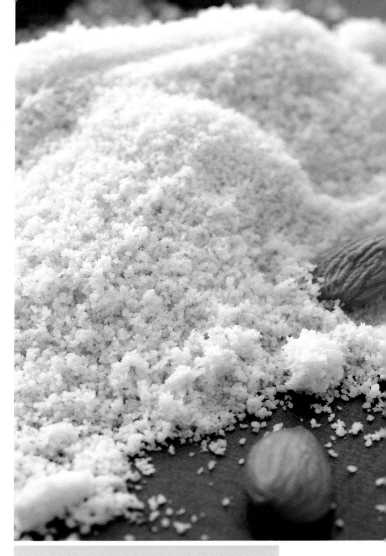

WHOLESOME AND GLUTEN-FREE

There are plenty of wholesome gluten-free alternatives. For baking bread try oat, coconut, or almond flour—they are all great substitutes. You can also choose rice, quinoa, oat kernels, buckwheat, legumes, potatoes, or root vegetables to ensure that your gluten-free diet is both nutritious and delicious.

47

Nature's Own Pantry

BALANCING BLOOD SUGAR NATURALLY

I hesitate to take just any kind of food supplement uncritically. Yet, far too many of us make a habit of swallowing pills and capsules without clearly understanding their effects and side effects. Seeking help for an ailment with alternative supplements that have a proven track record, however, is entirely different, and it's for that reason I will mention some foods and supplements that may actually help deal with elevated blood sugar.

Essentially, anything that can aid in reducing a diabetic person's dependence on traditional medication can only be beneficial: chromium, cinnamon, ALA, and fenugreek are some proven remedies we've already mentioned, but there are many more.

Milk thistle is a food supplement that also lowers blood sugar **(145)**, although it's mostly marketed as protection for the liver.

The sweet potato is a food that has blood sugar–lowering properties in addition to its nutritional advantage—its complex carbohydrates **(145)**.

Gooseberries have a blood sugar–lowering effect **(146)**. Freezing them won't diminish their effectiveness, either.

Some vegetables, such as bitter melon (Momordica charantia), contain potent blood sugar–lowering characteristics **(147)**.

SPICES THAT LOWER BLOOD SUGAR

There are several action mechanisms by which a spice can lower sugar levels in the blood. It can be, as is the case with cinnamon, a certain antioxidant that assists the cells in taking up glucose; there may also be substances that slow the breakdown of carbohydrates in the gastrointestinal tract.

Many spices have an inhibiting effect on amylase, an enzyme that works to break down starch into simple sugars in the mouth and in the small intestine. Black pepper is such a spice, as are ginger and garlic **(148)**. They slow down the digestive process, and this is reflected in the blood sugar curve. Starch must be broken down completely into glucose before it can be absorbed.

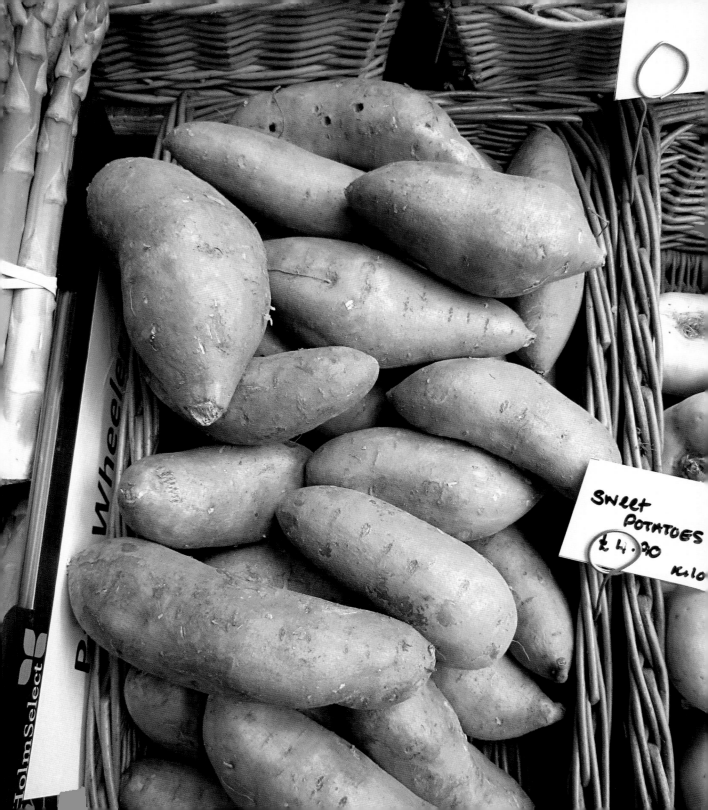

SWEET
POTATOES
£4.90
Kilo

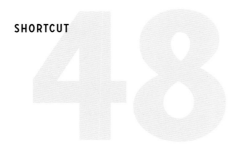

Sugar and Body Weight

SUGAR QUICKLY PACKS ON THE POUNDS

We all know that sugar contributes to weight gain, and that's probably why many of you have picked up this book. You want to rid yourself of sugar, the main cause of why you're carrying around more weight than you'd like.

Deep down it's easy to understand the mechanism. Your body needs a certain amount of nutrition to stay alive, and you obtain it through the food you eat.

Since sugar doesn't contribute any value to food except in pure carbohydrates and calories, it's just an add-on to what you have to eat in order to meet your true nutritional needs. Consuming a large amount of sugar means taking on surplus energy, which in time turns into that "spare tire" around your midsection.

To illustrate: eating an extra 100 calories per day over the course of a single year will pack on approximately 11 pounds of body fat! Those calories come from a mere 25 grams (1 ounce) of pure sugar—the amount you'd be getting from one piece of candy on your way home from work each day.

SUGAR TEACHES THE BODY TO STORE FAT

Our bodies have evolved over millions of years and have developed a finely honed skill to detect what we're eating. The body then adjusts its response depending on what we eat, choosing to utilize our food in specific ways.

When we consume sugar, the body will use that as fuel instead of using the fat we eat or have already stored. This means that when we eat sugar we send our body the message to store the fat and burn carbohydrates.

In response, the amount of enzymes that are responsible for producing body fat increases in our body. These lipogenic enzymes are needed to convert carbohydrates and protein into fat, and the more sugar we eat, the more of it will be converted into body fat **(149)**.

A further effect of eating large amounts of sugar is the decrease of the mitochondrial beta-oxidation enzymes. Beta-oxidation is the scientific term for fat burning within the body cells' power generators—the mitochondria.

FRUIT KEEPS YOU TRIM

We know that when foods taste sweet, they also make us feel good: the reward system is activated and sparks a large release of dopamine, while serotonin, which makes us happy and calm, is produced in the brain. Tasting sweet foods even prompts the release of endorphins, which makes them a real asset to life.

Endorphins are the body's own morphine, and they serve to calm us down, to quiet anxiety, and to relieve pain. As such, some sweetness in our food raises our enjoyment of life and makes us happy. It's only a question of getting the sweetness from the right source—that's where fruit comes in and refined sugar is kept at arm's length.

It's rumored in certain circles that fruit makes us fat and that we must avoid it as systematically as we do sugar. It's easy to fall for this theory, which asserts that it's the sweetness itself that makes us fat, and whether it comes from refined sugar or fruit is irrelevant.

However, there is a big difference between foods that are sweet in their natural, whole state, and something that has been artificially sweetened with high doses of refined sugar. There are 5 to 10 times as many fat-building calories in candy as there are in fruit—and remember that it's only the calories you don't use that will end up making you overweight. You need a certain amount of energy every day, and it's not the fruit in your diet that will cause a calorie surplus.

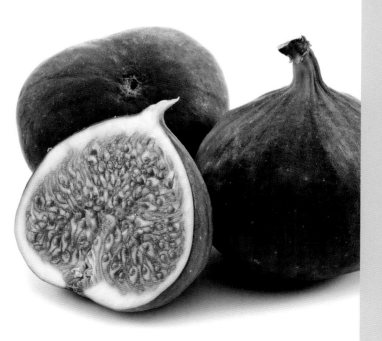

PEOPLE WHO EAT FRUIT WEIGH LESS

An extensive study was conducted at Harvard University to find the correlation between different foods and body weight. The research combed through all the literature on the subject of food and body weight, and the findings indicated that there was no danger of excess weight gain through fruit consumption. Not surprisingly, the study also showed that foods such as chips, soda, candy, and cookies were highly fattening. Even red meat was included in the group of unhealthy foods, while fish and dairy products were shown to keep us trim. As for fruit, its relationship to body fat appeared to be inversely correlated: people who ate the most fruit weighed the least, and vice versa.

THERE ARE 5 TO 10 TIMES AS MANY FAT-BUILDING **CALORIES IN CANDY** AS THERE ARE IN FRUIT. REMEMBER THAT IT'S ONLY THE CALORIES YOU DON'T USE THAT **WILL MAKE YOU OVERWEIGHT**.

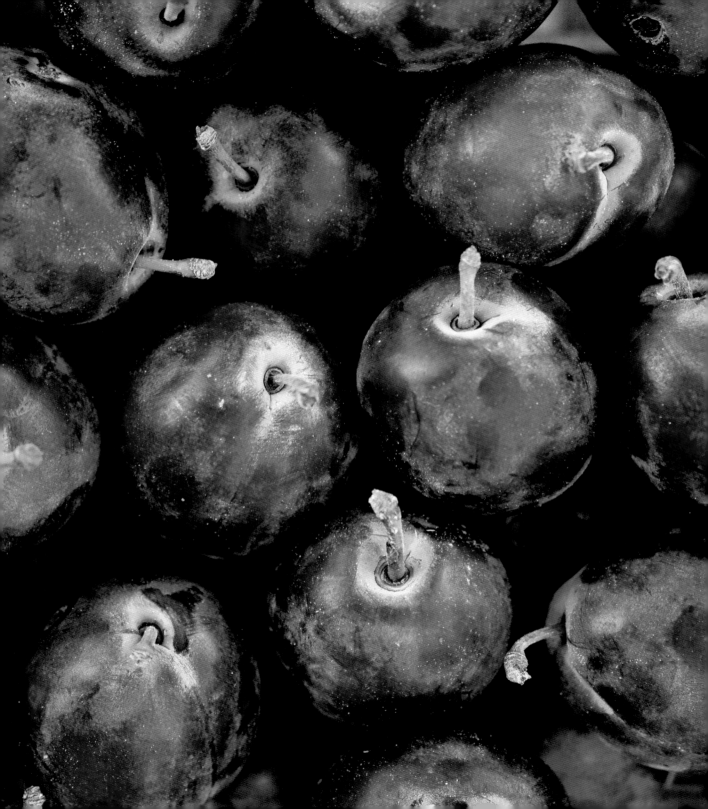

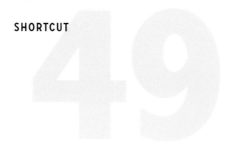

A Cool Down Lowers GI Value

A LOWER GI VALUE

A few years ago, it was observed that starchy foods like potatoes, rice, and pasta changed GI value after they were cooked and then cooled down. This happens because nutrients in cool food are stored by a different method, and glucose molecules bind differently. Some of the carbohydrates, instead of being easily digested as starch chains, become resistant starch, which results in the GI value and carbohydrate content decreasing and the fiber content increasing substantially. These are all good effects in many ways, with the added bonus that reheating the food does not return the starch to its former, easily digested starch chain incarnation. This means you can reheat yesterday's leftover brown rice or pasta for today's lunch and still keep its new, lower GI value.

How can we be sure that it's the resistant starch that's beneficial for blood sugar, and not just a general decrease in carbohydrate intake? We know because studies have shown that supplementing food with resistant starch decreases both insulin and blood sugar levels **(150)**. Likewise, foods with a high level of resistant starch give lower blood sugar responses in both healthy individuals **(151)** and in diabetics **(152)**.

THIS IS HOW RESISTANT STARCH WORKS

Resistant starch can be considered a hybrid of water-soluble and non-soluble fiber, as it contains beneficial properties belonging to both camps. Aside from in the aforementioned cooked and cooled foods, resistant starch can also be found in green (unripe) bananas, raw potatoes, and some types of corn. It's included in some breakfast cereal flakes and in breads. In truth, when white bread is marketed as "fiber-rich" even though it lacks whole meal flour, it's enriched with resistant starch. This is an improvement over its white, refined counterpart, despite the fact that the good nutrition provided by whole grains is still missing.

Generally speaking, it's healthy to eat resistant starch; I, myself, often prepare

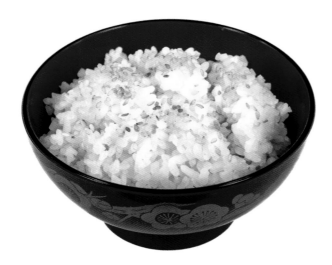

more rice, pasta, and potatoes than I need for one meal. The leftovers keep well in the refrigerator, and rice, in particular, is easy to freeze in single-size servings and defrost a few hours before it's time to eat. Since I always choose the most nutritious source of carbohydrates for my first meal, I know that any subsequent dish prepared with those leftovers will only be healthier.

RESISTANT STARCH AND WEIGHT CONTROL

The WHO (World Health Organization) considers the fiber content of food to be the strongest link to weight reduction

THE ADDITION OF RESISTANT STARCH LOWERS BOTH INSULIN AND BLOOD SUGAR.

(153). Resistant starch is of particular interest to food manufacturers, as it's a cheap ingredient and has a neutral taste.

Adding resistant starch to foods like breads, pastas, and energy bars is fine; naturally occurring resistant starch is equally beneficial.

When natural resistant starch is broken down in the large intestine you only get 2 or 3 calories per gram compared to the 4 calories you would get from fully digestible starch. This means that your blood sugar response will be much lower when you eat a meal high in resistant starch, which helps contribute to weight loss.

Naturally occurring resistant starch also seems to increase satiety after a meal (154, 155, 156), which in turn leads to lower calorie intake and thus, weight loss. Another interesting quality of resistant starch is that it has shown to increase the rate of fat burning after a meal (157). As it also decreases fat storage, resistant starch makes for an effective tool for anyone wanting to maintain low body fat (158).

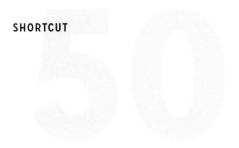

Enjoy a Good Coffee Break

A COFFEE BREAK IS IMPORTANT

A coffee break is invaluable. It gives us a small respite during the workday, as well as a chance to socialize with friends and colleagues. Workplaces that allow coffee breaks tend to work more efficiently, rather than suffer lost productivity. Staff morale is raised, and the pause encourages discussion about work topics and issues that might otherwise fall by the wayside due to lack of time.

The benefit of a coffee break is somewhat cancelled when cookies and pastries enter the picture. After the first sugar high takes effect, serotonin is released, which makes people feel tired and drowsy. Good work habits would be better served by having more suitable and sugar-free alternatives available to staff.

Some families and groups take coffee breaks every day, where it's easier to enjoy your own healthy snack. Things are trickier in the workplace, however.

One way to deal with this situation is to speak to the manager and request better food for the break room. If this isn't feasible, get a group of like-minded coworkers together and take turns bringing in sugar-free alternatives. It's likely that many others will find the healthier options tempting and want to join in. Oftentimes people feel pressured into sampling proffered sugary treats in order to not stick out or offend anyone, not because they want to eat the food. But a coffee break is a group activity, and as such you may as well make available healthy choices that do your body good.

WHICH COFFEE BREAK IS BEST?

To give credit where credit is due, I have to applaud the food manufacturer Delicato for their attention-grabbing ad campaign that showcases Swedish treats such as chocolate balls, snack cakes, and cookies. With slogans like "Guaranteed Free of Whole Grains" and "May Contain Traces of Vitamins and Minerals," they have effectively disarmed and won over those critical of their products. Irony is a very powerful weapon and I admire their chutzpah. Unfortunately, I need to focus on more nutritious fare for those who care about their health.

Most of us take a coffee break every day, and no one is going to feel up to the day's challenge if they eat lumps of sugar and unhealthy fat for a snack. If I feel like eating something on my break, I snap off a few squares of dark chocolate flavored with orange or mint. The taste is simultaneously sweet and bitter, which makes me feel satisfied after only a few bites.

It is well known that tart, bitter, and sour tastes inhibit appetite. This explains why the small amount of sugar I ingest does me little harm, while the large amount of antioxidants and minerals in my bit of chocolate will actually do me some good.

When I have a yen for something sweeter, I cut up a very sweet fruit like persimmon, watermelon, or orange. If they happen to be in season, they will taste their best and will definitely tame my craving for sugar. Even pomegranate goes well with coffee.

SUGAR-FREE COFFEE BREAK TREATS

Some people enjoy baking and making their own coffee break treats, and there is absolutely nothing wrong with this as long as they use the right ingredients.

These days, the Internet is teeming with recipes for sugar-free baked goods. In principle, opt for recipes that feature no added sugar and very small amounts of sifted, white wheat flour.

Flour shouldn't be of major concern, as long as other ingredients such as nuts, seeds, dried fruit, canola oil, coconut milk, almond flour, buckwheat, cottage cheese, buttermilk, or rye flour are included to bring down the GI value.

Honey is a good source of sweetness, but I believe the most popular sweetener for the baker who wants to avoid sugar is Sukrin (erythritol). Its popularity is based on the fact that erythritol shares many of the same qualities as sugar (see page 61).

TART, BITTER, AND SOUR TASTES INHIBIT APPETITE.

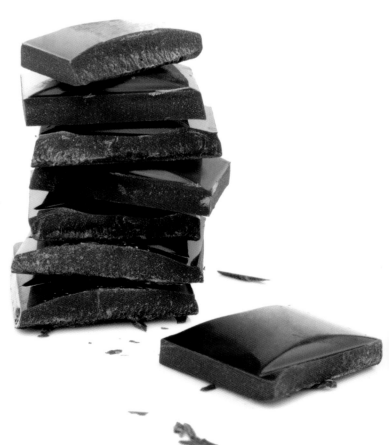

Endnotes

1 Landgren S, Simm JA, Thelle DS, Strandhagen E, Bartlett SE, Engel JA, Jerlhag E. *The ghrelin signalling system is involved in the consumption of sweets.* PLoS One. 2011 Mar 23;6(3):e18170.

2 Jakubowicz D, Froy O, Wainstein J, Boaz M. *Meal timing and composition influence ghrelin levels, appetite scores and weight loss maintenance in overweight and obese adults.* Steroids. 2012 Mar 10;77(4):323–31.

3 Bray G A. *Fructose and risk of cardiometabolic disease.* Curr Atheroscler Rep. 2012 Dec;14(6):570–8.doi:10.1007/s11883–012–0276–6.

4 Niinikoski H, Routtinen S. *Is carbohydrate intake in the first years of life related to future risk of NCDs?* Nutr Metab Cardiovasc Dis. 2012 Jul 10.

5 Eshak E S, Iso H, Mizoue T, Inoue M, Noda M, Tsugane S. *Soft drink, 100 percent fruit juice, and vegetable juice intakes and risk of diabetes mellitus.* Clin Nutr. 2012 Aug 13.

6 Attwood A S, Scott-Samuel NE, Stothart G, Munafò M R. *Glass shape influences consumption rate for alcoholic beverages.* PLoS One. 2012;7(8):e43007.doi:0.1371/journal.pone.0043007. Epub 2012 Aug 17.

7 Nseir W, Nassar F, Assy N. *Soft drinks consumption and nonalcoholic fatty liver disease.* World J Gastroenterol. 2010 Jun 7;16(21):2579–88.

8 Abid A, Taha O, Nseir W, Farah R, Grosovski M, Assy N. *Soft drink consumption is associated with fatty liver disease independent of metabolic syndrome.* J Hepatol. 2009 Nov;51(5):918–24. Epub 2009 Aug 21.

9 Assy N, Nasser G, Kamayse I, Nseir W, Beniashvili Z, Djibre A, Grosovski M. *Soft drink consumption linked with fatty liver in the absence of traditional risk factors.* Can J Gastroenterol. 2008 Oct;22(10):811–6.

10 Genkinger J M, Li R, Spiegelman D, Anderson K E, Albanes D, Bergkvist L, Bernstein L, Black A, van den Brandt P A, English D R, Freudenheim J L, Fuchs C S, Giles G G, Giovannucci E, Goldbohm R A, Horn-Ross P L, Jacobs E J, Koushik A, Männistö S, Marshall J R, Miller A B, Patel A V, Robien K, Rohan T E, Schairer C, Stolzenberg-Solomon R, Wolk A, Ziegler R G, Smith-Warner S A. *Coffee, tea and sugar-sweetened carbonated soft drink intake and pancreatic cancer risk: a pooled analysis of 14 cohort studies.* Cancer Epidemiol Biomarkers Prev. 2012 Feb;21(2):305–18. Epub 2011 Dec 22.

11 Mueller N T, Odegaard A, Anderson K, Yuan J M, Gross M, Koh W P, Pereira M A. *Soft drink and juice consumption and risk of pancreatic cancer: The Singapore Chinese Health Study.* Cancer Epidemiol Biomarkers Prev. 2010 Feb;19(2):447–55.

12 Englund-Ögge L, Brantsæter A L, Haugen M, Sengpiel V, Khatibi A, Myhre R, Myking S, Meltzer HM, Kacerovsky M, Nilsen RM, Jacobsson B. *Association between intake of artificially sweetened and sugar-sweetened beverages and preterm delivery: A large prospective cohort study.* Am J Clin Nutr. 2012 Sep;96(3):552–9.

13 de Konig L, Malik V S, Kellogg M D, Rimm E B, Willett W C, Hu F B. *Sweetened beverage consumption, incident coronary heart disease, and biomarkers of risk in men.* Circulation. 2012 Apr 10;125(14):1735–41.

14 Cohen L, Curhan G, Forman J. *Association of sweetened beverage intake with incident hypertension.* J Gen Intern Med. 2012 Sep;27(9):1127–34. Epub 2012 Apr 27.

15 Kristensen M, Jensen M, Kudsk J, Henriksen M, Mølgaard C. *Short-term effects on bone turnover of replacing milk with cola beverages: a 10-day interventional study in young men.* Osteoporos Int. 2005 Dec;16(12):1803–8. Epub 2005 May 11.

16 Jensdottir T, Arnadottir I B, Thorsdottir I, Bardow A, Gudmundsson K, Theodors A, Holbrook W P. *Relationship between dental erosion, soft drink consumption, and gastroesophageal reflux among Icelanders.* Clin Oral Investig. 2004 Jun;8(2):91–6. Epub 2004 Jan 27.

17 Saldana T M, Basso O, Darden R, Sandler D P. *Carbonated beverages and chronic kidney disease.* Epidemiology. 2007 Jul;18(4)501–6.

18 Belpoggi F, Soffritti M, Tibaldi E, Falcioni L, Bua L, Trabucco F. *Results of long-term carcinogenicity bioassays on Coca-Cola administered to Sprague-Radley rats.* Ann N Y Acad Sci. 2006 Sep;1076:736–52.

19 Malik V S, Schulze M B, Hu F B. *Intake of sugar-sweetened beverages and weight gain: A systematic review.* Am Clin Nutr. 2006 Aug;84(2):274–88.

20 Shang X W, Liu A L, Zhang Q, Hu X Q, Du S M, Ma J, Xu G F, Li Y, Guo H W, Du L, Li T Y, Ma G S. *Report on childhood obesity in China(9): Sugar-sweetened beverages consumption and obesity.* Biomed Environ Sci. 2012 Apr;25(2):125–32.

21 Jia M, Wang C, Zhang Y, Zheng Y, Zhang L, Huang Y, Wang P. *Sugary beverage intakes and obesity prevalence among junior high school students in Beijing—a cross-sectional research on SSBs intake.* Asia Pac J Clin Nutr. 2012;21(3):425–30.

22 Qi Q, Chu A Y, Kang J H, Jensen M K, Curhan G C, Pasquale L R, Ridker P M, Hunter D J, Willett W C, Rimm E B, Chasman D I, Hu F B, Qi L. *Sugar-sweetened beverages and genetic risk of obesity.* N Engl J Med, 2012 Oct 11;367(15):1387–96.

23 de Ruyter J C, Olthof M R, Seidell J C, Katan M B. *A trial of sugar-free or sugar-sweetened beverages and body weight in children.* N Engl J Med. 2012 Oct 11;367(15):1397–406.

24 Phillips K M, Carlsen M H, Blomhoff R. *Total antioxidant content of alternatives to refined sugar.* J Am Diet Assoc. 2009 Jan;109(1):64–71.

25 Hikosaka K, El-Abasy M, Koyama Y, Motobu M, Koge K, Isobe T, Kang C B, Hayashidani H, Onodera T, Wang P C, Matsumura M, Hirota Y. *Immunostimulating effects of the polyphenol-rich fraction of sugar cane* (Saccharum officinarum L) *extract in chickens.* Phytother Res. 2007 Feb;21(2):120–5.

26 Amer S, Na K J, Motobu M, El-Abasy M, Nakamura K, Koge K, Hirota Y.

Radioprotective effect of sugar cane in chickens. Phytother Res. 2005 Jun;19(6):496–500.

27 Holt S, Jong V D, Faramus E, Lang T, Brand Miller. *A bioflavonoid in sugar cane can reduce the postprandial glycaemic response to a high-GI starchy food.* J Asia Pac J Clin Nutr. 2003;12 Suppl:S66.

28 Bae Y J, Bak Y K, Kim B, Kim M S, Lee J H, Sung M K. *Coconut-derived D-xylose affects postprandial glucose and insulin responses in healthy individuals.* Nutr Res Pract. 2011 Dec;5(6):533–9.

29 Salil G, Nevin K G, Rajamohan T. *Arginine-rich coconut kernel diet influences nitric oxide synthase activity in alloxandiabetic rats.* J Sci Food Agric. 2012 Jul;92(9):1903–8.

30 Preetha P P, Devi V G, Rajamohan T. *Hypoglycemic and antioxidant potential of coconut water in experimental diabetes.* Food Funct. 2012 Jul;3(7):753–7.

31 Bhagya D, Prema L, Rajamohan T. *Therapeutic effects of tender coconut water on oxidative stress in fructose fed insulin resistant hypertensive rats.* Asian Pac J Trop Med. 2012 April;5(4):270–6.

32 Wiklund, A K, Breitholtz M, Bengtsson B E, Adolfsson-Erici M. *Sucralose— an ecotoxicological challenger?* Chemosphere. 2012 Jan;86(1):50–5. doi:10.1016/j.chemosphere.2011.08.049. Epub 2011 Sep 28.

33 *Products and Markets—Stevia.* Food and Agriculture Organization of the United Nations—Forestry Department. Retrieved 4 May 2007.

34 Goyal, S K, Samsher, Goyal R K. *Stevia (Stevia rebaudiana) a bio-sweetener: A review.* Int J Food Sci Nutr 61(1): 1–10. Feb 2010.

35 Anton S D, Martin C K, Han H, Coulon S, Cefalu W T, Geiselman P, Williamson D A. *Effects of stevia, aspartame, and sucrose on food intake, satiety, and postprandial glucose and insulin levels.* Appetite 55 (1):37–43. Aug 2010.

36 Blass E, Fitzgerald E, Kehoe P. *Interactions between sucralose, pain and isolation distress.* Pharmacol Biochem Behav. 1987 Mar; 26(3):483–9.

37 Avena N M, Rada P, Hoebel B G. *Evidence for sugar addiction; Behavioral and neurochemical effects of intermittent, excessive sugar intake.* Nerosci Biobehav Rev. 2008;32(1):20–39.

38 Burger K S, Stice E. *Frequent ice cream consumption is associated with reduced striatal response to* receipt of *an ice cream-based milkshake.* Am J Clin Nutr. 2012 Apr;95(4):810–7.

39 Phillips K M, Carlsen M H, Blomhoff R. *Total antioxidant content of alternatives to refined sugar.* J Am Diet Assoc. 2009 Jan;109(1):64–71.

40 Friberg E, Wallin A, Wolk A. *Sucrose, high-sugar foods, and risk of endometrial cancer—a population— based cohort study.* Cancer Epidemiol Biomarkers Prev. 2011 Sep;20(9):1831–7. Epub 2011 Jul 15.

41 Tasevska N, Jiao L, Cross A J, Kipnis V, Subar A F, Hollenbeck A, Schatzkin A, Potischman N. *Sugars in diet and risk of cancer in the NIH-AARP Diet and Health Study.* Int J Cancer. 2012 Jan 1;130(1):159–69. doi:10.1002/ijc.25990. Epub 2011 May 24.

42 Meinhold C L, Dodd K W, Jiao L, Flood A, Shikany J M, Genkinger J M, Hayes R B, Stolzenberg-Solomon R Z. *Available carbohydrates, glycemic load, and pancreatic cancer: Is there a link?* Am J Epidemiol. 2010 Jun 1;171(11):1174–82. Epub 2010 May 7.

43 Nöthlings U, Murphy S P, Wilkens L R, Henderson B E, Kolonel L N. *Dietary glycemic load, added sugars, and carbohydrates as risk factors for pancreatic cancer; The Multiethnic Cohort Study.* Am J Clin Nutr. 2007 Nov;86(5):1495–501.

44 Schernhammer E S, Hu F B, Giovannucci E, Michaud D S, Colditz G A, Stampfer M J, Fuchs C S. *Sugar-sweetened soft drink consumption and risk of pancreatic cancer in two prospective cohorts.* Cancer Epidemiol Biomarkers Prev. 2005 Sep;14(9):2098–105.

45 Aune D, Chan D S, Vieira A R, Navarro Rosenblatt D A, Vieira R, Greenwood D C, Cade J E, Burley V J, Norat T. *Dietary fructose, carbohydrates, glycemic indices and pancreatic cancer risk: A systematic review and meta-analysis of cohort studies.* Ann Oncol. 2012 Apr 26.

46 Hu J, La Vecchia C, Gibbons L, Negri E, Mery L. *Nutrients and risk of prostate cancer.* Nutr Cancer. 2010;62(6):710–8.

47 Bradshaw P T, Sagiv S K, Kabat G C, Satia J A, Britton J A, Teitelbaum S L, Neugut A I, Gammon M D. *Consumption of sweet foods and breast cancer risk: A case-control study of women in Long Island, New York.* Cancer Causes Control. 2009 Oct;20(8):1509–15. Epub 2009 April 23.

48 Hu J, La Vecchia C, DesMeules M, Negri E, Mery L. *Canadian Cancer Registries Epidemiology research Group. Nutrient and fiber intake and risk of renal cell carcinoma.* Nutr Cancer. 2008;60(6):720–8.

49 Michaud D S, Fuchs C S, Liu S, Willett W C, Colditz G A, Giovannucci E. *Dietary glycemic load, carbohydrate, sugar, and colorectal cancer risk in mean and women.* Cancer Epidemiol Biomarkers Prev. 2005 Jan;14(1):138–47.

50 Pfeiffer B, Stellingwerff T, Zaltas E, Jeukendrup A E. *CHO oxidation from a CHO gel compared with a drink during exercise.* Med Sci Sports Exerc. 2010 Nove;42(11):2038–45.

51 Brondel L, Romer M A, Nougues P M, Touyarou P, Davenne D. *Acute partial sleep deprivation increases food intake in healthy men.* Am J Clin Nutr. 2010 Jun;91(6):1550–9.

52 Knutson K L, Van Cauter E. *Associations between sleep loss and increased risk of obesity and diabetes.* Ann NY Acad Sci. 2008;1129:287–304.

53 Leproult R, Van Cauter E. *Role of sleep and sleep loss in hormonal release and metabolism.* Endocr Dev. 2010;17:11–21.

54 Schiavo-Cardozo D, Lima M M, Pareja J C, Geloneze B. *Appetite-regulating hormones from the upper gut: Disrupted control of xenin and ghrelin in night workers.* Clin Endocrinol (Oxf). 2012 Dec 1.

55 Gonnissen H K, Rutters F, Mazuy C, Martens E A, Adam T C, Westerterp-Plantenga M S. *Effect of a phase advance and phase delay of the 24-h cycle on energy metabolism, appetite, and related hormones.* Am J Clin Nutr. 2012 Oct;96(4):689–97. Epub 2012 Aug 22.

56 Hursel R, Rutters F, Gonnissen H K, Martens E A, Westerterp-Plantenga M S. *Effects of sleep fragmentation in healthy men on energy expenditure, substrate oxidation, physical activity, and exhaustion measured over 48 h in a respiratory chamber.* Am J Clin Nutr. 2011 Sep;94(3):804–8.

57 Blom W A, Lluch A, Stafleu A, Vinoy S, holst J J, Schaafsma G, Hendriks H F. *Effect of a high-protein breakfast on the postprandial ghrelin response.* Am J Clin Nutr. 2006 Feb;83(2):211–20.

58 Pérez-Torres I, Ruiz-Ramirez A, Baños G, El-Hafidi M. *Hibiscus Sabdariffa Linnaeus (Malvaceae), curcumin and resveratrol as alternative medicinal agents against metabolic syndrome.* Cardiovasc Hematol Agents Med Chem. 2012 Jun 20.

59 Enhörning S, Wang T J, Nilsson P M, Almgren P, Hedblad B, Berglund G, Struck J, Morgenthaler N G, Bergmann A, Lindholm E, Groop L, Lyssenko V, Orho-Melander M, Newton-Cheh C, Melander O. *Plasma copeptin and the risk of diabetes mellitus.* Circulation. 2010 May 18;121(19):2102–8.

60 Pan A, Malik V S, Schulze M B, Manson J E, Willett W C, Hu F B. *Plain-water intake and risk of type 2 diabetes in young and middle-aged women.* Am M Clin Nutr. 2012 Jun;95(6):1454–60.

61 Park S, Blanck H M, Sherry B, Brener N, O'Toole T. *Factors associated with low water intake among US high school students—National Youth Physical Activity and Nutrition Study, 2010.* J Acad Nutr Diet. 2012 Sep;112(9):1421–7.

62 Davy B M, Dennis E A, Dengo A L, Wilson K L, Day K P. *Water consumption reduces energy intake at a breakfast meal in obese older adults.* J Am Diet Assoc. 2008 Jul;108(7):1236–9.

63 Boschmann M, Steiniger J, Hille U et al. *Water-induced thermogenesis.* J. Clin Endocrinol Metab 2003;88:k6015–6019.

64 Stookey J D, Constant F, Popkin B M, Gardner C D. *Drinking water is associated with weight loss in overweight dieting women independent of diet and activity.* Obesity (Silver Spring). 2008 Nov;16(11):2481–8.

65 Watzek N, Scherbl D, Feld J, Berger F, Doroshyenko O, Fuhr U, Tomalik-Scharte D, Baum M, Eisenbrand G, Richling E. *Profiling of mercapturic acids of acrolein and acrylamide in humane urine after consumption of potato crisps.* Mol Nutr Food Res. 2012 Dec;56(12):1825–37.

66 Feng Z, Hu W, Hu Y, Tang M. *Acrolein is a major cigarette-related lung cancer agent: Preferential binding at p53 muttional hotspots and inhibition of DNA repair.* Proc Natl Acad Sci U S A. 2006 Oct 17;103(42):15404–9.

67 Kermani-Alghoraishi M, Anvari M, Talebi A R, Amini-Rad O, Ghahramani R, Miresmaili S M. *The effects of acrylamide on sperm parameters and membrane integrity of epididymal spermatozoa in mice.* Eur J Obstet Gynecol Reprod Biol. 2010 Nov;153(1):52–5.

68 El-Sayyad H I, Abou-Egla M H, El-Sayyad F I, El-Ghawet H A, Gaur R L, Fernando A, Raj M H, Ouhtit A. *Effects of fried potato chip supplementation on mouse pregnancy and fetal development.* Nutrtion. 2011 Mar;27(3):343–50.

69 Naruszewicz M, Zapolska-Downar D, Kosmider A, Nowicka G, Kozlowska-Wojciechowska M, Vikström A S, Törnqvist M. *Chronic intake of potato chips in humans increases the production of reactive oxygen radicals by leukocytes and increases plasma C-reactive protein: A pilot study.* Am J Clin Nutr. 2009 Mar;89(3):773–7.

70 Waegeneers N, Thiry C, De Temmerman L, Ruttens A. *Predicted dietary intake of selenium by the general adult population in Belgium.* Food Addit Contam Part A Chem Anal Control Expo Risk Assess. 2012 Nov 29.

71 Park K M, Fulgoni V L. *The association between dairy product consumption and cognitive function in the National Health and Nutrition Examination Survey.* Br J Nutr. 2012 Jul 24:1–8.

72 Høstmark A T, Haug A. *Does cheese intake blunt the association between soft drink intake and risk of the metabolic syndrome? Results from the cross-sectional Oslo Health Study.* BMJ Open. 2012 Nov 19;2(6).

73 Nguyen V, Cooper L, Lowndes J, Melanson K, Angelopoulos T J, Rippe J M, Reimers K. *Popcorn is more satiating than potato chips in normal-weight adults.* Nutr J. 2012 Sept14;11:71.

74 Strate L L, Liu Y L, Syngal S, Aldoori W H, Giovannucci E L. *Nut, corn, and popcorn consumption and the incidence of diverticular disease.* JAMA. 2008 Aug 27;300(8):907–14.

75 Martínez-González M A, Bes-Rastrollo M. *Nut consumption, weight gain and obesity; Epidemiological evidence.* Nutr Metab Cardiovasc Dis. 2011 Jun;21 Suppl 1:S40–5.

76 Vadivel V, Kunyanga C N, Bielsalski H K. *Health benefits of nut consumption with special reference to body weight control. Nutrition.* 2012 Nov–Dec;28(11–12):1089–97.

77 Mercanligil S M, Arslan P, Alasalvar C, Okut E, Akgül E, Pinar A, Geyik P O, Tokgözoğlu L, Shahidi F. *Effects of hazelnut-enriched diets on plasma cholesterol and lipoprotein profiles in hypercholesterolemic adult men.* Eur J Clin Nutr. 2007 Feb;61(2):212–20.

78 Yücesan F B, Orem A, Kural B V, Orem C, Turan I. *Hazelnut consumption decreases the susceptibility of LDL to oxidation, plasma oxidized LDL level and increases the ratio of large/small LDL in normolipidemic healthy subjects.* Anadoly Kardiyol Derg. 2010 Feb;10(1):28–35.

79 Simsek A, Aykut O. *Evaluation of the microelement profile of Turkish hazelnut (Corylus avellana L.) varities for human nutrition and health.* Int J Food Sci Nutr. 2007 Dec;58(8):677–88.

80. Cohen A E, Johnston C S. *Almond ingestion at mealtime reduces*

postprandial glycemia and chronic ingestion reduces hemoglobin A(1c) in individuals with well-controlled type 2 diabetes mellitus. Metabolism. 2011 Sep;60(9):1312–7.

81 Josse A R, Kendall C W. Augustin L S, Ellis P R, Jenkins D J. *Almonds and postprandial glycemia—a dose-response study.* Metabolism. 2007 Mar;56(3):400–4.

82 Griel A E, Cao Y, Bagshaw D D, Cifelli A M, Holub B, Kris-Etherton P M. *A macadamia-rich diet reduces total and LDL-cholesterol in mildly hypercholesterolemic men and women.* J Nutr. 2008 Apr;138(4):761–7.

83 Hudthagosol C, Haddad E, Jongsuwat R. *Antioxidant activity comparison of walnuts and fatty fish.* J Med Assoc Thai. 2012 Jun;95 Suppl 6:S179–88.

84 Casas-Agustench P, López-Uriarte P, Bulló M, Ros E, Cabré-Vila J J, Salas-Salvadó J. *Effects of one serving of mixed nuts on serum lipids, insulin resistance and inflammatory markers in patients with the metabolic syndrome.* Nutr metab Cardiovasc Dis. 2011 Feb;21(2):125–35.

85 Tapsell L C, Batterham M J, Teuss G, Tan S Y, Dalston S, Quick C J, Gillen L J, Charlton K E. *Long-term effects of increased dietary polyunsurared fat from walnuts on metabolic parameters in type II diabetes.* Eur J Clin Nutr. 2009 Aug;63(8):1008–15.

86 Ma Y, Njike V Y, Millet J, Dutta S, Doughty K, Treu J A, Katz D L. *Effects of walnut consumption on endothelial function in type 2 diabetic subjects: A randomized controlled crossover trial.* Diabetes Care. 2010 Feb;33(2);227–32.

87 Chandrasekara N, Shahidi F. *Effect of roasting on phenolic content and antioxidant activities of whole cashew nuts, kernels, and testa.* J Agric Food Chem. 2011 May 11;59(9):5006–14.

88 Reis C E, Bordalo L A, Rocha A L, Freitas D M, da Silva M V, de Faria V C, Martino H S, Costa N M, Alfenas R C. *Ground roasted peanuts leads to a lower post-prandial glycemic response than raw peanuts.* Nutr Hosp. 2011 Jul–Aug;26(4):745–51.

89 Bengmark S. *Diet of our time behind inflammation and disease development. Heating of food produces dysfunctional proteins which accumulates in the body.* Läkartidningen Nr 51–52, volume 104, pages 3873–3877, 2007.

90 Wang X, Li Z, Liu Y, Lv X, Yang W. *Effects of pistachios on body weight in Chinese subjects with metabolic syndrome.* Nutr J. 2012 Apr 3;11:20.

91 Kendall C W, Josse A R, Esfahani A, Jenkins D J. *The impact of pistachio intake alone or in combination with high-carbohydrate foods on postprandial glycemia.* Eur J Clin Nutr. 2011 Jun;65(6):696–702.

92 Kim S K, Karadeniz F. *Biological importance and applications of squalene and squalane.* Adv. Food Nutr Res. 2012;65:223-33l. doi:10.1016/B978-0-12-416003-3.00014-7.

93 Ryan E, Galvin K, O'Connor T P, Maguire A R, O'Brien N M. *Fatty acid profile, tocopherol, squalene and phytosterol content of brazil, pecan, pine, pistachio and cashew nuts.* Int J Food Sci Nutr. 2006 May–Jun;57(3–4):219–28.

94 McNay E C, Rechnagel A K. *Brain insulin signaling: A key component of cognitive processes and a potential basis for cognitive impairment in type 2 diabetes.* Neurobiol Learn Mem. 2011 Oct;96(3):432–42.

95 Sartorius T, Ketterer C, Kullmann S, Balzer M, Rotermund C, Binder S, Somoza V, Preissl H, Fritsche A, Häring H U, Henninge A M. *Monounsaturated fatty acids prevent the aversive effects of obesity on locomotion, brain activity, and sleep behavior.* Diabetes. 2012 Jul;61(7):1669–70.

96 Risérus U. *Fatty acids and insulin sensitivity.* Curr Opin Clin Nutr Metab Care. 2008 Mar;11(2):100–5.

97 Brennan I M, Luscombe-Marsh N D, Seimon R V, Otto B, Horowitz M, Wishart J M, Feinle-Bisset C. *Effects of fat, protein, and carbohydrates and protein load on appetite, plasma cholecystokinin, peptide YY, and ghrelin, and energy intake in lean and obese men.* Am J Physiol Gastrointest Liver Physiol. 2012 Jul;303(1):G129–40.

98 Brindal E, Baird D, Slater A, Danthiir V, Wilson C, Bowen J, Noakes M. *The effect of beverages varying in glycemic load on postprandial glucose response, appetite and cognition in 10–12-year-old school children.* Br J Nutr. 2012 Dec17:1–9.

99 Vikøren L A, Nygård O K, Lied E, Rostrup E, Gudbrandsen O A. *A randomized study on the effects of fish protein supplement on glucose tolerance, lipids and body composition in overweight adults.* Br J Nutr. 2012 May 31:1–10.

100 Leidy H J, Bales-Voelker L I, Harris C T. *A protein-rich beverage consumed as a breakfast meal leads to a weaker appetitive and dietary responses v. a protein-rich solid breakfast meal in adolescents.* Br J Nutr. 2011 Jul; 106(1):37–41.

101 Bengmark S. *Advanced glycation and lipoxidation end products—amplifiers of inflammation: The role of food.* JPEN Parenter Enteral Nutr 2007;31(S):430–40.

102 McConell G K, Rattigan S, Lee-Young R S, Wadley G D, Merry T L. *Skeletal muscle nitric oxide signaling and exercise: A focus on glucose metabolism.* Am J Physiol Endocrinol Metab. 2012 Aug1;303(3):E301–7.

103 Bird S R, Hawley J A. *Exercise and type 2 diabetes: new prescription for an old problem.* Maturitas. 2012 Aug;72(4):311–6.

104 Hoeks J, Schrauwen P. *Muscle mitochondria and insulin resistance: A human perspective.* Trends Endocrino Metab. 2012 Sep;23(9):444–50.

105 Wood R J, O'Neill E C. *Resistance training in type II diabetes mellitus: impact on areas of metabolic dysfunction in skeletal muscle and potential impact on bone.* J Nutr. Meta. 2012;2012:268197

106 Spadafranca A, Rinelli S, Riva A, Morazzoni P, Magni P, Bertoli S, Battezzati A. *Phaseolus vulgaris extract affects glycometabolic and appetite control in healthy human subjects.* Br J Nutr. 2012 Oct 9:1–7.

107 Spreadbury I. *Comparison with ancestral diets suggests dense acellular carbohydrates promote an inflammatory microbiota, and may be the primary dietary cause of leptin* resistance and obesity. Diabetes Metab Syndr Obes. 2012;5:175–89.

108 Kosova E C, Auinger P, Bremer A A. *The relationships between sugar-sweetened beverage intake and cardio-metabolic markers in young children.* J Acad Nutr Diet. 2013 Feb;113(2):219–27.

109 Kwon H H, Yoon J Y, Hong J S, Jung J Y, Park M S, Suh D H. *Clinical and histological effect of a low glycaemic load diet in treatment of acne vulgaris in Korean patients: A randomized, controlled trial.* Acta Derm Venereol. 2012 May;92(3):241–6.

110 Buyken A E, Flood V, Empson M, Rochtchina E, Barclay A W, Brand-Miller J, Mitchell P. *Carbohydrate nutrition and inflammatory disease mortality in older adults.* Am J Clin Nutr. 2010 Sep;92(3):634–43.

111 Magistrelli A. Chezem J C. *Effect of ground cinnamon on postprandial blood glucose concentration in normal-weight and obese adults.* J Acad Nutr Diet. 2012 Nov;112(11):1806–9.

112 Hlebowicz J, Hlebowicz A, Lindstedt S, Björgell O, Höglund P, Holst J J, Darwiche G, Almér L O. *Effects of 1 and 3 g cinnamon on gastric emptying, satiety, and postprandial blood glucose, insulin, glucose-dependent insulinotropic polypeptide, glucagon-like peptide 1, and ghrelin concentrations in healthy subjects.* Am J Clin Nutr. 2009 Mar;89(3):815–21.

113 Hlebowicz J, Darwiche G, Björgell O, Almér L O. *Effect of cinnamon on postprandial blood glucose, gastric emptying, and satiety in healthy subjects.* Am J Clin Nutr. 2007 Jun;85(6):1552–6.

114 Davis P A, Yokoyama W. *Cinnamon intake lowers fasting blood glucose: meta-analysis.* J Med Food. 2011 Sep;14(9):884–9.

115 Vafa M, Mohammadi F, Shidfar F, Sormaghi M S, Heidari I, Golestan B, Amiri F. *Effects of cinnamon consumption on glycemic status, lipid profile and body composition in type 2 diabetic patients.* Int J Prev Med. 2012 Aug;3(8):531–6.

116 Zhou J, Chan L, Zhou S. *Trigonelline: A plant alkaloid with therapeutic*

potential for diabetes and central nervous system disease. Curr Med Chem. 2012;19(21).

117 Puri D, Prabhu K M, Dev G, Agarwal S, Murthy P S. *Mechanism of antidiabetic action of compound GII purified from fenugreek (Trigonella foenum graecum) seeds.* Indian J Clin Biochem 2011 Oct;26(4):335–46.

118 Gutierres V O, Pinheiro C M, Assis R P, Vendramini R C, Pepato M T, Brunetti I L. *Curcumin-supplemented yoghurt improves physiological and biochemical markers of experimental diabetes.* Br J Nutr. 2012 Aug;108(3):440–8.

119 Na L X, Zhang Y L, Li Y, Liu L Y, Li R, Kong T, Sun C H. *Curcumin improves insulin resistance in skeletal muscle of rats.* Nutr Metab Cardiovasc Dis. 2011 Jul;21(7):526–33.

120 Whitehead N, White H. *Systematic review of randomised controlled trials to the effects of caffeine or caffeinated drinks on blood glucose concentrations and insulin sensitivity in people with diabetes mellitus.* J Hum Nutr Diet. 2013 Jan 19.

121 Bassoli B K, Cassolla P, Borba-Murad G R, Constantin J, Salgueiro-Pagadigorria C L, Bazotte R B, da Silva R S, de Souza H M. *Chlorogenic acid reduces the plasma glucose peak in the oral glucose tolerance test: effects on hepatic glucose release and glycaemia.* Cell Biochem Funct. 2007 Nov 7.

122 Iso H, Date C, Wakai K, Fukui M, Tamakoshi A; JACC Study Group. *The relationship between green tea and total caffeine intake and risk for self-reported type 2 diabetes among Japanese adults.* Ann Intern Med. 2006 Apr 18;144(8):554–62.

123 Panagiotakos D B, Lionis C, Zeimbekis A, Makri K, Bountziouka V, Economou M, Vlachou I, Micheli M, Tsakountakis N, Metallinos G, Polychronopoulos E. *Long-term, moderate coffee consumption is associated with lower prevalence of diabetes mellitus among elderly non-tea drinkers from the Mediterranean Islands (MEDIS Study).* Rev Diabet Stud. 2007 Summer;4(2):105–11.

124 van Dijk A E, Olthof M R, Meeuse J C, Seebus E, Heine R J, van Dam R M.

Acute effects of decaffeinated coffee and the major coffee components chlorogenic acid and trigonelline on glucos tolerance. Diabetes Care. 2009 Jun;32(6):1023–5.

125 Yamashita Y, Wang L, Tinshun Z, Nakamura T, Ashida H. *Fermented tea improves glucose intolerance in mice by enhancing translocation of glucose transporter 4 in skeletal muscle.* J Agric Food Chem. 2012 Nov 14;60(45):11366–71.

126 Schöttker B, Herder C, Rothenbacher D, Perna L, Müller H, Brenner H. *Serum 25-hydroxyvitamin D levels and incident diabetes mellitus tupe 2: A competing risk analysis in a large population-based cohort of older adults.* Eur J Epidemiol 2013 Jan 26.

127 Afzal S, Bojesen S E, Nordestgaard B G. *Low 25-hydroxyvitamin D and risk of type 2 diabetes: A prospective cohort study and metaanalysis.* Clin Chem 2013 Feb;59(2):381–91.

128 Soheilykhah S, Mojibian M, Moghadam M J, Shojaoddiny-Ardekani A. *The effect of different doses of vitamin D supplementation on insulin resistance during pregnancy.* Gynecol Endocrinol. 2013 Jan 25.

129 Ross A C, Taylor C L, Yaktine A L, et al. *8, implications and special concerns. Institute of Medicine (US) Committee to review dietary reference intakes for vitamin D and calcium (2011).* Dietary Reference Intakes for Calcium and Vitamin D. Washington DC: National Academies Press. ISBN 0–309–16394–3.

130 Lankinen M, Schwab U, Kolehmainen M, Paananen J, Poutanen K, mykkänen H, Seppänen-Laakso T, Gylling H, Uusitupa M, Orešič M. *Whole grain products, fish and bilberries alter glucose and lipid metabolism in a randomized, controlled trial: The Sysdimet study.* PLoS One. 2011;6(8).

131 Jang Y, Lee J H, Kim O Y, Park H Y, Lee S Y. *Consumption of whole grain and legume powder reduces insulin demand, lipid peroxidation, and plasma homocysteine concentration in patients with coronary artery disease: randomized controlled clinical* trial. Arterioscler Throb Vasc Biol 2001 Dec;21(12):2065–71.

132 Wirström T, Hilding A, Gu H F, Ostenson C G, Björklund A. *Consumption of whole grain reduces risk of deteriorating glucose tolerance, including progression to prediabetes.* Am J Clin Nutr. 2013 Jan;97(1):179–87.

133 Bartlomiej S, Justyna R K, Ewa N. *Bioactive compounds in cereal grains—occurrence, structure, technological significance and nutritional benefits—a review.* Food Sci Technol Int. 2012 Dec;18(6):559–68.

134 Lefevre M, Jonnalagadda S. *Effect of whole grains on markers of subclinical inflammation.* Nutr Rev. 2012 Dec;18(6):559–68.

135 Rasoamanana R, Chaumontet C, Nadkarni N, Tomé D, Fromentin G, Darcel N. *Dietary fibers solubilized in water or an oil emulsion induce satiation through CCK-mediated vagal signaling in mice.* J Nutr. 2012 Nov;142(11):2033–9.

136 Mani U V, Mani I, Biswas M, Kumar S N. *An open-label study on the effect of flax seed powder (Linum usitatissimum) supplementation in the management of diabetes mellitus.* J Diet Suppl 2011 Sep;8(3):257–65.

137 Park Y, Subar A F, Hollenbeck A, Schatzkin A. *Dietary fiber intake and mortality in the NIH-AARP Diet and Health Study.* Arch Intern Med 171(12):1061–8, Feb 14, 2011.

138 Udupa A S, Nahar P S, Shah S H, Kshirsagar M J, Ghongane B B. *Study of comparative effects of antioxidants on insulin sensitivity in type 2 diabetes mellitus.* J Clin Diagn Res 2012 Nov;6(9):1469–73.

139 Castro M C, Massa M L, Schinella G, Gagliardino J J, Francini F. *Lipoic acid prevents liver metabolic changes induced by administration of a fructose-rich diet.* Biochim Biophys Acta. 2013 Jan;1830(1):2226–32.

140 Han T, Bai J, Liu W, Hu Y. *A systematic review and meta-analysis of alpha-lipoic acid in the treatment of diabetic peripheral neuropathy.* Eur J Endocrinol. 2012 Oct;167(4):465–71.

141 Harding S V, Rideout T C, Jones P J. *Evidence for using alpha-lipoic acid in reducing lipoprotein and inflammatory related atherosclerotic risk.* J Diet Suppl. 2012 Jun;9(2):116–27.

142 Porasuphatana S, Suddee S, Nartnampong A, Konsil J, Harnwong B, Santaweesuk A. *Glycemic and oxidative status of patients with type 2 diabetes mellitus following oral administration of alpha-lipoic acid: a randomized double-blinded placebo-controlled study.* Asia Pac J Clin Nutr. 2012;21(1):12–21.

143 Masharani U, Gjerde C, McCoy S, Maddux B A, Hessler D, Goldfine I D, Youngren J F. *Chromium supplementation in non-obese non-diabetic subjects is associated with a decline in insulin sensitivity.* BMC Endocr Disord. 2012 Nov 30;12(1):31.

144 Ouellet V, Marois J, Weisnagel S J, Jacques H. *Dietary cod protein improves insulin sensitivity in insulin-resistant men and women: A randomized controlled trial.* Diabetes Care. 2007 Nov;30(11):2816–21.

145 Suksomboon N, Poolsup N, Boonkaew S, Suthisisang C C. *Meta-analysis of the effect of herbal supplement on glycemic control in type 2 diabetes.* J Ethnopharmacol. 2011 Oct11; 137(3):1378–33.

146 Deng R. *A review of the hypoglycemic effects of five commonly used herbal food supplements.* Recent Pat Food Nutr Agric. 2012 Apr1;4(1):50–60.

147 Chaturvedi P. *Antidiabetic potentials of Momordica charantia: multiple mechanisms behind the effects.* J Med Food. 2012 Feb;15(2):101–7.

148 P S Zinjarde S S, Bhargava S Y, Kumar A R. *Potent α-amylase inhibitory activity of Indian Ayurvedic medicinal plants.* BMC Complement Altern Med. 2011 Jan 20;11:5.

149 Sartor F, Jackson M J, Squillace C, Shepherd A, Moore J P, Ayer D E, Kubis H P. *Adaptive metabolic response to 4 weeks of sugar-sweetened beverage consumption in healthy, lightly active individuals and chronic high glucose availability in primary human myotubes.* Eur J Nutr. 2012 June 26.

150 Klosterbuer A S, Thomas W, Slavin J L. *Resistant starch and pullulan reduce postprandial glucose, insulin, and GLP-1, but have no effect on satiety in healthy humans.* J Agric Food Chem. 2012 Dec5;60(48):11928–34.

151 Vonk R J, Hagedoorn R E, de Graaff R et al. *Digestion of so-called resistant starch sources in the human small intestine.* Am. J. Clin. Nutr. 72 (2): 432–8. Aug 2000.

152 Giacco R, Clemente G, Brighenti F, Mancini M, Coppola S, Ruffa G, Rivieccio A M, Rivellese A, Riccardi G et al. *Metabolic effects of resistant starch in patients with type 2 diabetes.* Diab Nutr Metab 1998 (11):330–335.

153 World Health Organization, Joint WHO/FAO Expert Consultation. *Diet, Nutrition and the Prevention of Chronic Diseases.* 2003, WHO Technical Report Series 916.

154 Anderson G H, Cho C E, Akhavan T, Mollard R C, Luhovyy B L, Finocchiaro E T. *Relation between estimates of cornstarch digestibility by the Englyst in vitro method and glycemic response, subjective appetite, and short-term food intake in young men.* Am J Clin Nutr. 2010 Apr;91(4):932-9. doi:10.3945/ajcn.2009.28443. Epub 2010 Feb 17.

155 Bodinham C L, Frost G S, Roberson M D. *Acute ingestion of resistant starch reduces food intake in healthy adults.* Br J Nutr. 2010 Mar;103(6):917-22. doi:10.1017/S0007114509992534. Epub 2009 Oct 27.

156 Nilsson A C, Ostman E M, Holst J J, Björck I M. *Including indigestible carbohydrates in the evening meal of healthy subjects improves glucose tolerance, lowers inflammatory markers, and increases satiety after a subsequent standardized breakfast.* J Nutr. 2008 Apr;138(4):732-9.

157 Higgins J A, Higbee D R, Donahoo W T, Brown I L, Bell M L, Bessesen D H. *Resistant starch consumption promotes lipid oxidation.* Nutr Metab (Lond). 2004 Oct 6;1(1):8.

158 Robertson M D, Wright J W, Loizon E, Debard C, Vidal H, Shojaee-Moradie F, Russell-Jones D, Umpleby A M. *Insulin-sensitizing effects on muscle and adipose tissue after dietary fiber intake in men and women with metabolic syndrome.* J. Clin Endocrinol Metab. 2012.

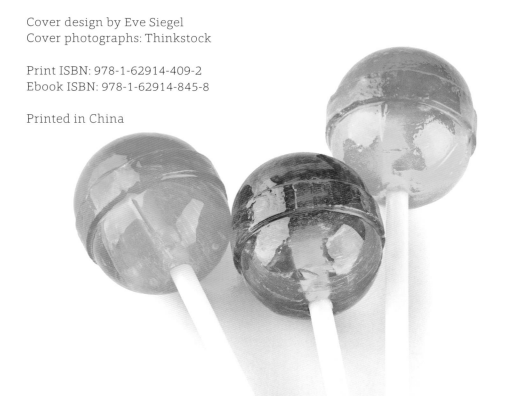